D0848767

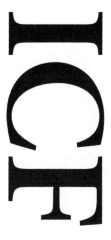

International Classification of Functioning, Disability and Health

World Health Organization
Geneva

WHO Library Cataloguing-in-Publication Data

International classification of functioning, disability and health : ICF.

1.Human development 2.Body constitution 3. Health status 4. Disability
evaluation 5.Socioeconomic factors 6.Causality 7.Classification 8.Manuals
I.Title: ICF

(ISBN 92 4 154542 9)   (NLM classification: W 15)

Contents

ICF

Introduction

1. Background

This volume contains the *International Classification of Functioning, Disability and Health,* known as ICF.[1] The overall aim of the ICF classification is to provide a unified and standard language and framework for the description of health and health-related states. It defines components of health and some health-related components of well-being (such as education and labour). The domains contained in ICF can, therefore, be seen as *health domains* and *health-related domains.* These domains are described from the perspective of the body, the individual and society in two basic lists: (1) Body Functions and Structures; and (2) Activities and Participation.[2] As a classification, ICF systematically groups different domains[3] for a person in a given health condition (e.g. what a person with a disease or disorder does do or can do). *Functioning* is an umbrella term encompassing all body functions, activities and participation; similarly, *disability* serves as an umbrella term for impairments, activity limitations or participation restrictions. ICF also lists environmental factors that interact with all these constructs. In this way, it enables the user to record useful profiles of individuals' functioning, disability and health in various domains.

ICF belongs to the "family" of international classifications developed by the World Health Organization (WHO) for application to various aspects of health. The WHO family of international classifications provides a framework to code a wide range of information about health (e.g. diagnosis, functioning and disability, reasons for contact with health services) and uses a standardized common language permitting communication about health and health care across the world in various disciplines and sciences.

In WHO's international classifications, health conditions (diseases, disorders, injuries, etc.) are classified primarily in ICD-10 (shorthand for the International

---

[1] The text represents a revision of the International Classification of Impairments, Disabilities, and Handicaps (ICIDH), which was first published by the World Health Organization for trial purposes in 1980. Developed after systematic field trials and international consultation over the past five years, it was endorsed by the Fifty-fourth World Health Assembly for international use on 22 May 2001 (resolution WHA54.21).

[2] These terms, which replace the formerly used terms "impairment", "disability" and "handicap", extend the scope of the classification to allow positive experiences to be described. The new terms are further defined in this Introduction and are detailed within the classification. It should be noted that these terms are used with specific meanings that may differ from their everyday usage.

[3] A domain is a practical and meaningful set of related physiological functions, anatomical structures, actions, tasks, or areas of life.

Classification of Diseases, Tenth Revision),[4] which provides an etiological framework. Functioning and disability associated with health conditions are classified in ICF. ICD-10 and ICF are therefore complementary,[5] and users are encouraged to utilize these two members of the WHO family of international classifications together. ICD-10 provides a "diagnosis" of diseases, disorders or other health conditions, and this information is enriched by the additional information given by ICF on functioning.[6] Together, information on diagnosis plus functioning provides a broader and more meaningful picture of the health of people or populations, which can then be used for decision-making purposes.

The WHO family of international classifications provides a valuable tool to describe and compare the health of populations in an international context. The information on mortality (provided by ICD-10) and on health outcomes (provided by ICF) may be combined in summary measures of population health for monitoring the health of populations and its distribution, and also for assessing the contributions of different causes of mortality and morbidity.

ICF has moved away from being a "consequences of disease" classification (1980 version) to become a "components of health" classification. "Components of health" identifies the constituents of health, whereas "consequences" focuses on the impacts of diseases or other health conditions that may follow as a result. Thus, ICF takes a neutral stand with regard to etiology so that researchers can draw causal inferences using appropriate scientific methods. Similarly, this approach is also different from a "determinants of health" or "risk factors" approach. To facilitate the study of determinants or risk factors, ICF includes a list of environmental factors that describe the context in which individuals live.

---

[4] International Statistical Classification of Diseases and Related Health Problems, Tenth Revision, Vols. 1-3. Geneva, World Health Organization, 1992-1994.

[5] It is also important to recognize the overlap between ICD-10 and ICF. Both classifications begin with the body systems. Impairments refer to body structures and functions, which are usually parts of the "disease process" and are therefore also used in the ICD-10. Nevertheless, ICD-10 uses impairments (as signs and symptoms) as parts of a constellation that forms a "disease", or sometimes as reasons for contact with health services, whereas the ICF system uses impairments as problems of body functions and structures associated with health conditions.

[6] Two persons with the same disease can have different levels of functioning, and two persons with the same level of functioning do not necessarily have the same health condition. Hence, joint use enhances data quality for medical purposes. Use of ICF should not bypass regular diagnostic procedures. In other uses, ICF may be used alone.

4

2. Aims of ICF

ICF is a multipurpose classification designed to serve various disciplines and different sectors. Its specific aims can be summarized as follows:

- to provide a scientific basis for understanding and studying health and health-related states, outcomes and determinants;

- to establish a common language for describing health and health-related states in order to improve communication between different users, such as health care workers, researchers, policy-makers and the public, including people with disabilities;

- to permit comparison of data across countries, health care disciplines, services and time;

- to provide a systematic coding scheme for health information systems.

These aims are interrelated, since the need for and uses of ICF require the construction of a meaningful and practical system that can be used by various consumers for health policy, quality assurance and outcome evaluation in different cultures.

2.1   Applications of ICF

Since its publication as a trial version in 1980, ICIDH has been used for various purposes, for example:

- as a statistical tool – in the collection and recording of data (e.g. in population studies and surveys or in management information systems);

- as a research tool – to measure outcomes, quality of life or environmental factors;

- as a clinical tool – in needs assessment, matching treatments with specific conditions, vocational assessment, rehabilitation and outcome evaluation;

- as a social policy tool – in social security planning, compensation systems and policy design and implementation;

- as an educational tool – in curriculum design and to raise awareness and undertake social action.

Since ICF is inherently a health and health-related classification it is also used by sectors such as insurance, social security, labour, education, economics, social policy and general legislation development, and environmental modification. It has been accepted as one of the United Nations social classifications and is referred to in and incorporates *The Standard Rules on the Equalization of*

Opportunities for Persons with Disabilities.[7] Thus ICF provides an appropriate instrument for the implementation of stated international human rights mandates as well as national legislation.

ICF is useful for a broad spectrum of different applications, for example social security, evaluation in managed health care, and population surveys at local, national and international levels. It offers a conceptual framework for information that is applicable to personal health care, including prevention, health promotion, and the improvement of participation by removing or mitigating societal hindrances and encouraging the provision of social supports and facilitators. It is also useful for the study of health care systems, in terms of both evaluation and policy formulation.

---

[7] *The Standard Rules on the Equalization of Opportunities for Persons with Disabilities.* Adopted by the United Nations General Assembly at its 48th session on 20 December 1993 (resolution 48/96). New York, NY, United Nations Department of Public Information, 1994.

3.   Properties of ICF

A classification should be clear about what it classifies: its universe, its scope, its units of classification, its organization, and how these elements are structured in terms of their relation to each other. The following sections explain these basic properties of ICF.

3.1 Universe of ICF

ICF encompasses all aspects of human health and some health-relevant components of well-being and describes them in terms of *health domains* and *health-related domains.*[*] The classification remains in the broad context of health and does not cover circumstances that are not health-related, such as those brought about by socioeconomic factors. For example, because of their race, gender, religion or other socioeconomic characteristics people may be restricted in their execution of a task in their current environment, but these are not health-related restrictions of participation as classified in ICF.

There is a widely held misunderstanding that ICF is only about people with disabilities; in fact, it is about *all people.* The health and health-related states associated with all health conditions can be described using ICF. In other words, ICF has universal application.[*]

3.2 Scope of ICF

ICF provides a description of situations with regard to human functioning and its restrictions and serves as a framework to organize this information. It structures the information in a meaningful, interrelated and easily accessible way.

ICF organizes information in two parts. Part 1 deals with Functioning and Disability, while Part 2 covers Contextual Factors. Each part has two components:

1. Components of Functioning and Disability

The **Body** component comprises two classifications, one for functions of body systems, and one for body structures. The chapters in both classifications are organized according to the body systems.

---

[*] Examples of health domains include seeing, hearing, walking, learning and remembering, while examples of health-related domains include transportation, education and social interactions.

[*] Bickenbach JE, Chatterji S, Badley EM, Üstün TB. Models of disablement, universalism and the ICIDH, *Social Science and Medicine*, 1999, 48:1173-1187.

The **Activities and Participation** component covers the complete range of domains denoting aspects of functioning from both an individual and a societal perspective.

2. Components of Contextual Factors

A list of **Environmental Factors** is the first component of Contextual Factors. Environmental factors have an impact on all components of functioning and disability and are organized in sequence from the individual's most immediate environment to the general environment.

Personal Factors is also a component of Contextual Factors but they are not classified in ICF because of the large social and cultural variance associated with them.

The components of Functioning and Disability in Part 1 of ICF can be expressed in two ways. On the one hand, they can be used to indicate problems (e.g. impairment, activity limitation or participation restriction summarized under the umbrella term *disability*); on the other hand they can indicate nonproblematic (i.e. neutral) aspects of health and health-related states summarized under the umbrella term *functioning).*

These components of functioning and disability are interpreted by means of four separate but related *constructs*. These constructs are operationalized by using *qualifiers*. Body functions and structures can be interpreted by means of changes in physiological systems or in anatomical structures. For the Activities and Participation component, two constructs are available: *capacity* and *performance* (see section 4.2).

A person's functioning and disability is conceived as a dynamic interaction[10] between health conditions (diseases, disorders, injuries, traumas, etc.) and contextual factors. As indicate above, Contextual Factors include both personal and environmental factors. ICF includes a comprehensive list of environmental factors as an essential component of the classification. Environmental factors interact with all the components of functioning and disability. The basic construct of the Environmental Factors component is the facilitating or hindering impact of features of the physical, social and attitudinal world.

3.3 Unit of classification

ICF classifies health and health-related states. The unit of classification is, therefore, *categories* within health and health-related domains. It is important to note, therefore, that in ICF persons are not the units of classification; that is, ICF does not classify people, but describes the situation of each person within an array of health or health-related domains. Moreover, the description is always made within the context of environmental and personal factors.

---

[10] This interaction can be viewed as a *process* or a *result* depending on the user.

3.4 Presentation of ICF

ICF is presented in two versions in order to meet the needs of different users for varying levels of detail.

The *full version* of ICF, as contained in this volume, provides classification at four levels of detail. These four levels can be aggregated into a higher-level classification system that includes all the domains at the second level. The two-level system is also available as a *short version* of ICF.

4.   Overview of ICF components

DEFINITIONS[11]

In the context of health:

Body functions are the physiological functions of body systems (including psychological functions).

Body structures are anatomical parts of the body such as organs, limbs and their components.

Impairments are problems in body function or structure such as a significant deviation or loss.

Activity is the execution of a task or action by an individual.

Participation is involvement in a life situation.

Activity limitations are difficulties an individual may have in executing activities.

Participation restrictions are problems an individual may experience in involvement in life situations.

Environmental factors make up the physical, social and attitudinal environment in which people live and conduct their lives.

An overview of these concepts is given in Table 1; they are explained further in operational terms in section 5.1. As the table indicates:

- ICF has two *parts*, each with two *components:*

    Part 1. Functioning and Disability
    - (a) Body Functions and Structures
    - (b) Activities and Participation

    Part 2. Contextual Factors
    - (c) Environmental Factors
    - (d) Personal Factors

- Each component can be expressed in both *positive* and *negative* terms.

- Each component consists of various domains and, within each domain, categories, which are the units of classification. Health and health-related states of an individual may be recorded by selecting the appropriate category

---

[11] See also Annex 1, Taxonomic and Terminological Issues.

code or codes and then adding *qualifiers*, which are numeric codes that specify the extent or the magnitude of the functioning or disability in that category, or the extent to which an environmental factor is a facilitator or barrier.

Table 1. An overview of ICF

	Part 1: Functioning and Disability		Part 2: Contextual Factors	
Components	Body Functions and Structures	Activities and Participation	Environmental Factors	Personal Factors
Domains	Body functions Body structures	Life areas (tasks, actions)	External influences on functioning and disability	Internal influences on functioning and disability
Constructs	Change in body functions (physiological) Change in body structures (anatomical)	Capacity Executing tasks in a standard environment Performance Executing tasks in the current environment	Facilitating or hindering impact of features of the physical, social, and attitudinal world	Impact of attributes of the person
Positive aspect	Functional and structural integrity *Functioning*	Activities Participation	Facilitators	not applicable
Negative aspect	Impairment *Disability*	Activity limitation Participation restriction	Barriers / hindrances	not applicable

4.1 Body Functions and Structures and impairments

Definitions: **Body functions** *are the physiological functions of body systems (including psychological functions).*

Body structures *are anatomical parts of the body such as organs, limbs and their components.*

Impairments *are problems in body function or structure as a significant deviation or loss.*

(1) Body functions and body structures are classified in two different sections. These two classifications are designed for use in parallel. For example, body functions include basic human senses such as "seeing functions" and their structural correlates exist in the form of "eye and related structures".

(2) "Body" refers to the human organism as a whole; hence it includes the brain and its functions, i.e. the mind. Mental (or psychological) functions are therefore subsumed under body functions.

(3) Body functions and structures are classified according to body systems; consequently, body structures are not considered as organs.[12]

(4) Impairments of structure can involve an anomaly, defect, loss or other significant deviation in body structures. Impairments have been conceptualized in congruence with biological knowledge at the level of tissues or cells and at the subcellular or molecular level. For practical reasons, however, these levels are not listed.[13] The biological foundations of impairments have guided the classification and there may be room for expanding the classification at the cellular or molecular levels. For medical users, it should be noted that impairments are not the same as the underlying pathology, but are the manifestations of that pathology.

(5) Impairments represent a deviation from certain generally accepted population standards in the biomedical status of the body and its functions, and definition of their constituents is undertaken primarily by those qualified to judge physical and mental functioning according to these standards.

(6) Impairments can be temporary or permanent; progressive, regressive or static; intermittent or continuous. The deviation from the population norm may be slight or severe and may fluctuate over time. These characteristics are captured in further descriptions, mainly in the codes, by means of qualifiers after the point.

---

[12] Although organ level was mentioned in the 1980 version of ICIDH, the definition of an "organ" is not clear. The eye and ear are traditionally considered as organs; however, it is difficult to identify and define their boundaries, and the same is true of extremities and internal organs. Instead of an approach by "organ", which implies the existence of an entity or unit within the body, ICF replaces this term with "body structure".

[13] Thus impairments coded using the full version of ICF should be detectable or noticeable by others or the person concerned by direct observation or by inference from observation.

12

(7) Impairments are not contingent on etiology or how they are developed; for
     example, loss of vision or a limb may arise from a genetic abnormality or an
     injury. The presence of an impairment necessarily implies a cause; however,
     the cause may not be sufficient to explain the resulting impairment. Also,
     when there is an impairment, there is a dysfunction in body functions or
     structures, but this may be related to any of the various diseases, disorders or
     physiological states.

(8) Impairments may be part or an expression of a health condition, but do not
     necessarily indicate that a disease is present or that the individual should be
     regarded as sick.

(9) Impairments are broader and more inclusive in scope than disorders or
     diseases; for example, the loss of a leg is an impairment of body structure,
     but not a disorder or a disease.

(10) Impairments may result in other impairments; for example, a lack of muscle
     power may impair movement functions, heart functions may relate to deficit
     in respiratory functions, and impaired perception may relate to thought
     functions.

(11) Some categories of the Body Functions and Structures component and the
     ICD-10 categories seem to overlap, particularly with regard to symptoms
     and signs. However, the purposes of the two classifications are different.
     ICD-10 classifies symptoms in special chapters to document morbidity or
     service utilization, whereas ICF shows them as part of the body functions,
     which may be used for prevention or identifying patients' needs. Most
     importantly, in ICF the Body Functions and Structures classification is
     intended to be used along with the Activities and Participation categories.

(12) Impairments are classified in the appropriate categories using defined
     identification criteria (e.g. as present or absent according to a threshold
     level). These criteria are the same for body functions and structures. They
     are: (a) loss or lack; (b) reduction; (c) addition or excess; and (d) deviation.
     Once an impairment is present, it may be scaled in terms of its severity using
     the generic qualifier in the ICF.

(13) Environmental factors interact with body functions, as in the interactions
     between air quality and breathing, light and seeing, sounds and hearing,
     distracting stimuli and attention, ground texture and balance, and ambient
     temperature and body temperature regulation.

4.2 Activities and Participation /activity limitations and participation restrictions

Definitions: *Activity is the execution of a task or action by an individual.*

Participation is involvement in a life situation.

Activity limitations are difficulties an individual may have in executing activities.

Participation restrictions are problems an individual may experience in involvement in life situations.

(1)   The domains for the Activities and Participation component are given in a *single list* that covers the full range of life areas (from basic learning or watching to composite areas such as interpersonal interactions or employment). The component can be used to denote activities (a) or participation (p) or both. The domains of this component are qualified by the two qualifiers of *performance* and *capacity*. Hence the information gathered from the list provides a data matrix that has no overlap or redundancy (see Table 2).

Table 2. Activities and Participation: information matrix

Domains		Qualifiers	
		Performance	Capacity
d1	Learning and applying knowledge		
d2	General tasks and demands		
d3	Communication		
d4	Mobility		
d5	Self-care		
d6	Domestic life		
d7	Interpersonal interactions and relationships		
d8	Major life areas		
d9	Community, social and civic life		

(2) The *performance* qualifier describes what an individual does in his or her current environment. Because the current environment includes a societal context, performance can also be understood as "involvement in a life situation" or "the lived experience" of people in the actual context in which they live.[14] This context includes the environmental factors – all aspects of the physical, social and attitudinal world which can be coded using the Environmental Factors component.

(3) The *capacity* qualifier describes an individual's ability to execute a task or an action. This construct aims to indicate the highest probable level of functioning that a person may reach in a given domain at a given moment. To assess the full ability of the individual, one would need to have a "standardized" environment to neutralize the varying impact of different environments on the ability of the individual. This standardized environment may be: (a) an actual environment commonly used for capacity assessment in test settings; or (b) in cases where this is not possible, an assumed environment which can be thought to have a uniform impact. This environment can be called a "uniform" or "standard" environment. Thus, capacity reflects the environmentally adjusted ability of the individual. This adjustment has to be the same for all persons in all countries to allow for international comparisons. The features of the uniform or standard environment can be coded using the Environmental Factors classification. The gap between capacity and performance reflects the difference between the impacts of current and uniform environments, and thus provides a useful guide as to what can be done to the environment of the individual to improve performance.

(4) Both capacity and performance qualifiers can further be used with and without assistive devices or personal assistance. While neither devices nor personal assistance eliminate the impairments, they may remove limitations on functioning in specific domains. This type of coding is particularly useful to identify how much the functioning of the individual would be limited without the assistive devices (see coding guidelines in Annex 2)

(5) Difficulties or problems in these domains can arise when there is a qualitative or quantitative alteration in the way in which an individual carries out these domain functions. *Limitations* or *restrictions* are assessed against a generally accepted population standard. The standard or norm against which an individual's capacity and performance is compared is that of an individual without a similar health condition (disease, disorder or injury, etc.). The limitation or restriction records the discordance between the observed and the expected performance. The expected performance is the population norm, which represents the experience of people without the specific health

---

[14] The definition of "participation" brings in the concept of involvement. Some proposed definitions of "involvement" incorporate taking part, being included or engaged in an area of life, being accepted, or having access to needed resources. Within the information matrix in Table 2 the only possible indicator of participation is coding through performance. This does not mean that participation is automatically equated with performance. The concept of involvement should also be distinguished from the subjective experience of involvement (the sense of "belonging"). Users who wish to code involvement separately should refer to the coding guidelines in Annex 2.

condition. The same norm is used in the capacity qualifier so that one can infer what can be done to the environment of the individual to enhance performance.

(6) A problem with performance can result directly from the social environment, even when the individual has no impairment. For example, an individual who is HIV-positive without any symptoms or disease, or someone with a genetic predisposition to a certain disease, may exhibit no impairments or may have sufficient capacity to work, yet may not do so because of the denial of access to services, discrimination or stigma.

(7) It is difficult to distinguish between "Activities" and "Participation" on the basis of the domains in the Activities and Participation component. Similarly, differentiating between "individual" and "societal" perspectives on the basis of domains has not been possible given international variation and differences in the approaches of professionals and theoretical frameworks. Therefore, ICF provides a single list that can be used, if users so wish, to differentiate activities and participation in their own operational ways. This is further explained in Annex 3. There are four possible ways of doing so:

  (a) to designate some domains as activities and others as participation, not allowing any overlap;

  (b) same as (a) above, but allowing partial overlap;

  (c) to designate all detailed domains as activities and the broad category headings as participation;

  (d) to use all domains as both activities and participation.

4.3 Contextual Factors

Contextual Factors represent the complete background of an individual's life and living. They include two components: Environmental Factors and Personal Factors – which may have an impact on the individual with a health condition and that individual's health and health-related states.

Environmental factors make up the physical, social and attitudinal environment in which people live and conduct their lives. These factors are external to individuals and can have a positive or negative influence on the individual's performance as a member of society, on the individual's capacity to execute actions or tasks, or on the individual's body function or structure.

(1) Environmental factors are organized in the classification to focus on two different levels:

  (a) *Individual* – in the immediate environment of the individual, including settings such as home, workplace and school. Included at this level are the physical and material features of the environment that an individual comes face to face with, as well as direct contact with others such as family, acquaintances, peers and strangers.

16

(b) *Societal* – formal and informal social structures, services and overarching approaches or systems in the community or society that have an impact on individuals. This level includes organizations and services related to the work environment, community activities, government agencies, communication and transportation services, and informal social networks as well as laws, regulations, formal and informal rules, attitudes and ideologies.

(2) Environmental factors interact with the components of Body Functions and Structures and Activities and Participation. For each component, the nature and extent of that interaction may be elaborated by future scientific work. Disability is characterized as the outcome or result of a complex relationship between an individual's health condition and personal factors, and of the external factors that represent the circumstances in which the individual lives. Because of this relationship, different environments may have a very different impact on the same individual with a given health condition. An environment with barriers, or without facilitators, will restrict the individual's performance; other environments that are more facilitating may increase that performance. Society may hinder an individual's performance because either it creates barriers (e.g. inaccessible buildings) or it does not provide facilitators (e.g. unavailability of assistive devices).

Personal factors are the particular background of an individual's life and living, and comprise features of the individual that are not part of a health condition or health states. These factors may include gender, race, age, other health conditions, fitness, lifestyle, habits, upbringing, coping styles, social background, education, profession, past and current experience (past life events and concurrent events), overall behaviour pattern and character style, individual psychological assets and other characteristics, all or any of which may play a role in disability at any level. Personal factors are not classified in ICF. However, they are included in Fig. 1 to show their contribution, which may have an impact on the outcome of various interventions.

5. Model of Functioning and Disability

5.1 Process of functioning and disability

As a classification, ICF does not model the "process" of functioning and disability. It can be used, however, to describe the process by providing the means to map the different constructs and domains. It provides a multi-perspective approach to the classification of functioning and disability as an interactive and evolutionary process. It provides the building blocks for users who wish to create models and study different aspects of this process. In this sense, ICF can be seen as a language: the texts that can be created with it depend on the users, their creativity and their scientific orientation. In order to visualize the current understanding of interaction of various components, the diagram presented in Fig. 1 may be helpful.[15]

Fig. 1. Interactions between the components of ICF

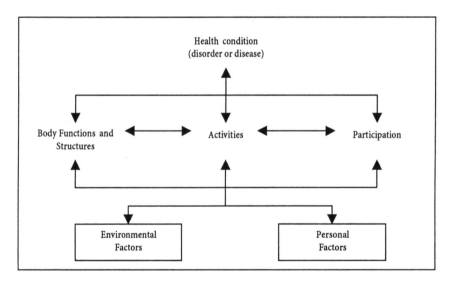

---

[15] ICF differs substantially from the 1980 version of ICIDH in the depiction of the interrelations between functioning and disability. It should be noted that any diagram is likely to be incomplete and prone to misrepresentation because of the complexity of interactions in a multidimensional model. The model is drawn to illustrate multiple interactions. Other depictions indicating other important foci in the process are certainly possible. Interpretations of interactions between different components and constructs may also vary (for example, the impact of environmental factors on body functions certainly differs from their impact on participation).

In this diagram, an individual's functioning in a specific domain is an interaction or complex relationship between the health condition and contextual factors (i.e. environmental and personal factors). There is a dynamic interaction among these entities: interventions in one entity have the potential to modify one or more of the other entities. These interactions are specific and not always in a predictable one-to-one relationship. The interaction works in two directions; the presence of disability may even modify the health condition itself. To infer a limitation in capacity from one or more impairments, or a restriction of performance from one or more limitations, may often seem reasonable. It is important, however, to collect data on these constructs independently and thereafter explore associations and causal links between them. If the full health experience is to be described, all components are useful. For example, one may:

- have impairments without having capacity limitations (e.g. a disfigurement in leprosy may have no effect on a person's capacity);

- have performance problems and capacity limitations without evident impairments (e.g. reduced performance in daily activities associated with many diseases);

- have performance problems without impairments or capacity limitations (e.g. an HIV-positive individual, or an ex-patient recovered from mental illness, facing stigmatization or discrimination in interpersonal relations or work);

- have capacity limitations without assistance, and no performance problems in the current environment (e.g. an individual with mobility limitations may be provided by society with assistive technology to move around);

- experience a degree of influence in a reverse direction (e.g. lack of use of limbs can cause muscle atrophy; institutionalization may result in loss of social skills).

Case examples in Annex 4 further illustrate possibilities of interactions between the constructs.

The scheme shown in Fig. 1 demonstrates the role that contextual factors (i.e. environmental and personal factors) play in the process. These factors interact with the individual with a health condition and determine the level and extent of the individual's functioning. Environmental factors are extrinsic to the individual (e.g. the attitudes of the society, architectural characteristics, the legal system) and are classified in the Environmental Factors classification. Personal Factors, on the other hand, are not classified in the current version of ICF. They include gender, race, age, fitness, lifestyle, habits, coping styles and other such factors. Their assessment is left to the user, if needed.

5.2 Medical and social models

A variety of conceptual models[16] has been proposed to understand and explain disability and functioning. These may be expressed in a dialectic of "medical model" versus "social model". The *medical model* views disability as a problem of the person, directly caused by disease, trauma or other health condition, which requires medical care provided in the form of individual treatment by professionals. Management of the disability is aimed at cure or the individual's adjustment and behaviour change. Medical care is viewed as the main issue, and at the political level the principal response is that of modifying or reforming health care policy. The *social model* of disability, on the other hand, sees the issue mainly as a socially created problem, and basically as a matter of the full integration of individuals into society. Disability is not an attribute of an individual, but rather a complex collection of conditions, many of which are created by the social environment. Hence the management of the problem requires social action, and it is the collective responsibility of society at large to make the environmental modifications necessary for the full participation of people with disabilities in all areas of social life. The issue is therefore an attitudinal or ideological one requiring social change, which at the political level becomes a question of human rights. For this model disability is a political issue.

ICF is based on an integration of these two opposing models. In order to capture the integration of the various perspectives of functioning, a "biopsychosocial" approach is used. Thus, ICF attempts to achieve a synthesis, in order to provide a coherent view of different perspectives of health from a biological, individual and social perspective.[17]

---

[16] The term "model" here means construct or paradigm, which differs from the use of the term in the previous section.

[17] See also Annex 5 - "ICF and people with disabilities".

6. Use of ICF

ICF is a classification of human functioning and disability. It systematically groups health and health-related domains. Within each component, domains are further grouped according to their common characteristics (such as their origin, type, or similarity) and ordered in a meaningful way. The classification is organized according to a set of principles (see Annex 1). These principles refer to the interrelatedness of the levels and the hierarchy of the classification (sets of levels). However, some categories in ICF are arranged in a non-hierarchical manner, with no ordering but as equal members of a branch.

The following are structural features of the classification that have a bearing on its use.

(1) ICF gives standard operational definitions of the health and health-related domains as opposed to "vernacular" definitions of health. These definitions describe the essential attributes of each domain (e.g. qualities, properties, and relationships) and contain information as to what is included and excluded in each domain. The definitions contain commonly used anchor points for assessment so that they can be translated into questionnaires. Conversely, results from existing assessment instruments can be coded in ICF terms. For example, "seeing functions" are defined in terms of functions of sensing form and contour, from varying distances, using one or both eyes, so that the severity of difficulties of vision can be coded at mild, moderate, severe or total levels in relation to these parameters.

(2) ICF uses an alphanumeric system in which the letters b, s, d and e are used to denote Body Functions, Body Structures, Activities and Participation, and Environmental Factors. These letters are followed by a numeric code that starts with the chapter number (one digit), followed by the second level (two digits), and the third and fourth levels (one digit each).

(3) ICF categories are "nested" so that broader categories are defined to include more detailed subcategories of the parent category. (For example, Chapter 4 in the Activities and Participation component, on Mobility, includes separate categories on standing, sitting, walking, carrying items, and so on). The short (concise) version covers two levels, whereas the full (detailed) version extends to four levels. The short version and full version codes are in correspondence, and the short version can be aggregated from the full version.

(4) Any individual may have a range of codes at each level. These may be independent or interrelated.

(5) The ICF codes are only complete with the presence of a *qualifier*, which denotes a magnitude of the level of health (e.g. severity of the problem). Qualifiers are coded as one, two or more numbers after a point (or *separator*). Use of any code should be accompanied by at least one qualifier. Without qualifiers, codes have no inherent meaning.

(6)   The first qualifier for Body Functions and Structures, the performance and capacity qualifiers for Activities and Participation, and the first qualifier for Environmental Factors all describe the extent of problems in the respective component.

(7)   All three components classified in ICF (Body Functions and Structures, Activities and Participation, and Environmental Factors) are quantified using the same generic scale. Having a problem may mean an impairment, limitation, restriction or barrier depending on the construct. Appropriate qualifying words as shown in brackets below should be chosen according to the relevant classification domain (where xxx stands for the second-level domain number). For this quantification to be used in a universal manner, assessment procedures need to be developed through research. Broad ranges of percentages are provided for those cases in which calibrated assessment instruments or other standards are available to quantify the impairment, capacity limitation, performance problem or barrier. For example, when "no problem" or "complete problem" is specified the coding has a margin of error of up to 5%. "Moderate problem" is defined as up to half of the time or half the scale of total difficulty. The percentages are to be calibrated in different domains with reference to relevant population standards as percentiles.

xxx.0 NO problem	(none, absent, negligible,…)	0-4 %
xxx.1 MILD problem	(slight, low,…)	5-24 %
xxx.2 MODERATE problem	(medium, fair,...)	25-49 %
xxx.3 SEVERE problem	(high, extreme, …)	50-95 %
xxx.4 COMPLETE problem	(total,…)	96-100 %
xxx.8 not specified		
xxx.9 not applicable		

(8)   In the case of environmental factors, this first qualifier can be used to denote either the extent of positive effects of the environment, i.e. facilitators, or the extent of negative effects, i.e. barriers. Both use the same 0-4 scale, but to denote facilitators the point is replaced by a plus sign: for example e110+2. Environmental Factors can be coded (a) in relation to each construct individually, or (b) overall, without reference to any individual construct. The first option is preferable, since it identifies the impact and attribution more clearly.

(9)   For different users, it might be appropriate and helpful to add other kinds of information to the coding of each item. There are a variety of additional qualifiers that could be useful. Table 3 sets out the details of the qualifiers for each component as well as suggested additional qualifiers to be developed.

(10) The descriptions of health and health-related domains refer to their use at a given moment (i.e. as a snapshot). However, use at multiple time points is possible to describe a trajectory over time and process.

(11) In ICF, a person's health and health-related states are given an array of codes that encompass the two parts of the classification. Thus the maximum

number of codes per person can be 34 at the one-digit level (8 body functions, 8 body structures, 9 performance and 9 capacity codes). Similarly, for the two-level items the total number of codes is 362. At more detailed levels, these codes number up to 1424 items. In real-life applications of ICF, a set of 3 to 18 codes may be adequate to describe a case with two-level (three-digit) precision. Generally the more detailed four-level version is used for specialist services (e.g. rehabilitation outcomes, geriatrics), whereas the two-level classification can be used for surveys and clinical outcome evaluation.

Further coding guidelines are presented in Annex 2. Users are strongly recommended to obtain training in the use of the classification through WHO and its network of collaborating centres.

Table 3. Qualifiers

Components	First qualifier	Second qualifier
Body Functions (b)	Generic qualifier with the negative scale used to indicate the extent or magnitude of an impairment Example: b167.3 to indicate a severe impairment in specific mental functions of language	None
Body Structures (s)	Generic qualifier with the negative scale used to indicate the extent or magnitude of an impairment Example: s730.3 to indicate a severe impairment of the upper extremity	Used to indicate the nature of the change in the respective body structure: 0 no change in structure 1 total absence 2 partial absence 3 additional part 4 aberrant dimensions 5 discontinuity 6 deviating position 7 qualitative changes in structure, including accumulation of fluid 8 not specified 9 not applicable Example: s730.32 to indicate the partial absence of the upper extremity
Activities and Participation (d)	Performance Generic qualifier Problem in the person's current environment Example: d5101.1_ to indicate mild difficulty with bathing the whole body with the use of assistive devices that are available to the person in his or her current environment	Capacity Generic qualifier Limitation without assistance Example: d5101._2 to indicate moderate difficulty with bathing the whole body; implies that there is moderate difficulty without the use of assistive devices or personal help
Environmental Factors (e)	Generic qualifier, with negative and positive scale, to denote extent of barriers and facilitators respectively Example: e130.2 to indicate that products for education are a moderate barrier. Conversely, e130+2 would indicate that products for education are a moderate facilitator	None

54th World Health Assembly endorsement of ICF for international use

The resolution WHA54.21 reads as follows:

The Fifty-fourth World Health Assembly,

1.   ENDORSES the second edition of the International Classification of Impairments, Disabilities and Handicaps (ICIDH), with the title International Classification of Functioning, Disability and Health, henceforth referred to in short as ICF;

2.   URGES Member States to use ICF in their research, surveillance and reporting as appropriate, taking into account specific situations in Member States and, in particular, in view of possible future revisions;

3.   REQUESTS the Director-General to provide support to Member States, at their request, in making use of ICF.

ICF

One-Level Classification

List of chapter headings in the classification

Body functions

Chapter 1	Mental functions
Chapter 2	Sensory functions and pain
Chapter 3	Voice and speech functions
Chapter 4	Functions of the cardiovascular, haematological, immunological and respiratory systems
Chapter 5	Functions of the digestive, metabolic and endocrine systems
Chapter 6	Genitourinary and reproductive functions
Chapter 7	Neuromusculoskeletal and movement-related functions
Chapter 8	Functions of the skin and related structures

Body structures

Chapter 1	Structures of the nervous system
Chapter 2	The eye, ear and related structures
Chapter 3	Structures involved in voice and speech
Chapter 4	Structures of the cardiovascular, immunological and respiratory systems
Chapter 5	Structures related to the digestive, metabolic and endocrine systems
Chapter 6	Structures related to the genitourinary and reproductive systems
Chapter 7	Structures related to movement
Chapter 8	Skin and related structures

Activities and participation

Chapter 1   Learning and applying knowledge

Chapter 2   General tasks and demands

Chapter 3   Communication

Chapter 4   Mobility

Chapter 5   Self-care

Chapter 6   Domestic life

Chapter 7   Interpersonal interactions and relationships

Chapter 8   Major life areas

Chapter 9   Community, social and civic life

Environmental factors

Chapter 1   Products and technology

Chapter 2   Natural environment and human-made changes to environment

Chapter 3   Support and relationships

Chapter 4   Attitudes

Chapter 5   Services, systems and policies

ICF

Two-Level classification

List of chapter headings
and first branching level
in the classification

BODY FUNCTIONS

Chapter 1 Mental functions

Global mental functions (b110-b139)

b110   Consciousness functions
b114   Orientation functions
b117   Intellectual functions
b122   Global psychosocial functions
b126   Temperament and personality functions
b130   Energy and drive functions
b134   Sleep functions
b139   Global mental functions, other specified and unspecified

Specific mental functions (b140-b189)

b140   Attention functions
b144   Memory functions
b147   Psychomotor functions
b152   Emotional functions
b156   Perceptual functions
b160   Thought functions
b164   Higher-level cognitive functions
b167   Mental functions of language
b172   Calculation functions
b176   Mental function of sequencing complex movements
b180   Experience of self and time functions
b189   Specific mental functions, other specified and unspecified
b198   Mental functions, other specified
b199   Mental functions, unspecified

Chapter 2 Sensory functions and pain

Seeing and related functions (b210-b229)

b210   Seeing functions
b215   Functions of structures adjoining the eye
b220   Sensations associated with the eye and adjoining structures
b229   Seeing and related functions, other specified and unspecified

Hearing and vestibular functions (b230-b249)

b230   Hearing functions
b235   Vestibular functions
b240   Sensations associated with hearing and vestibular function
b249   Hearing and vestibular functions, other specified and unspecified

Additional sensory functions (b250-b279)

b250   Taste function
b255   Smell function
b260   Proprioceptive function
b265   Touch function
b270   Sensory functions related to temperature and other stimuli

b279   Additional sensory functions, other specified and unspecified

Pain (b280-b289)
b280   Sensation of pain
b289   Sensation of pain, other specified and unspecified
b298   Sensory functions and pain, other specified
b299   Sensory functions and pain, unspecified

Chapter 3 Voice and speech functions
b310   Voice functions
b320   Articulation functions
b330   Fluency and rhythm of speech functions
b340   Alternative vocalization functions
b398   Voice and speech functions, other specified
b399   Voice and speech functions, unspecified

Chapter 4 Functions of the cardiovascular, haematological, immunological and respiratory systems

Functions of the cardiovascular system (b410-b429)
b410   Heart functions
b415   Blood vessel functions
b420   Blood pressure functions
b429   Functions of the cardiovascular system, other specified and unspecified

Functions of the haematological and immunological systems (b430-b439)
b430   Haematological system functions
b435   Immunological system functions
b439   Functions of the haematological and immunological systems, other
       specified and unspecified

Functions of the respiratory system (b440-b449)
b440   Respiration functions
b445   Respiratory muscle functions
b449   Functions of the respiratory system, other specified and unspecified

Additional functions and sensations of the cardiovascular and respiratory systems (b450-b469)
b450   Additional respiratory functions
b455   Exercise tolerance functions
b460   Sensations associated with cardiovascular and respiratory functions
b469   Additional functions and sensations of the cardiovascular and respiratory
       systems, other specified and unspecified
b498   Functions of the cardiovascular, haematological, immunological and
       respiratory systems, other specified
b499   Functions of the cardiovascular, haematological, immunological and
       respiratory systems, unspecified

Chapter 5 Functions of the digestive, metabolic and endocrine systems

Functions related to the digestive system (b510-b539)

b510 Ingestion functions
b515 Digestive functions
b520 Assimilation functions
b525 Defecation functions
b530 Weight maintenance functions
b535 Sensations associated with the digestive system
b539 Functions related to the digestive system, other specified and unspecified

Functions related to metabolism and the endocrine system (b540-b559)

b540 General metabolic functions
b545 Water, mineral and electrolyte balance functions
b550 Thermoregulatory functions
b555 Endocrine gland functions
b559 Functions related to metabolism and the endocrine system, other specified and unspecified
b598 Functions of the digestive, metabolic and endocrine systems, other specified
b599 Functions of the digestive, metabolic and endocrine systems, unspecified

Chapter 6 Genitourinary and reproductive functions

Urinary functions (b610-b639)

b610 Urinary excretory functions
b620 Urination functions
b630 Sensations associated with urinary functions
b639 Urinary functions, other specified and unspecified

Genital and reproductive functions (b640-b679)

b640 Sexual functions
b650 Menstruation functions
b660 Procreation functions
b670 Sensations associated with genital and reproductive functions
b679 Genital and reproductive functions, other specified and unspecified
b698 Genitourinary and reproductive functions, other specified
b699 Genitourinary and reproductive functions, unspecified

Chapter 7 Neuromusculoskeletal and movement-related functions

Functions of the joints and bones (b710-b729)

b710 Mobility of joint functions
b715 Stability of joint functions
b720 Mobility of bone functions
b729 Functions of the joints and bones, other specified and unspecified

Muscle functions (b730-b749)

b730 Muscle power functions
b735 Muscle tone functions
b740 Muscle endurance functions
b749 Muscle functions, other specified and unspecified

Movement functions (b750-b789)

b750 Motor reflex functions
b755 Involuntary movement reaction functions
b760 Control of voluntary movement functions
b765 Involuntary movement functions
b770 Gait pattern functions
b780 Sensations related to muscles and movement functions
b789 Movement functions, other specified and unspecified
b798 Neuromusculoskeletal and movement-related functions, other specified
b799 Neuromusculoskeletal and movement-related functions, unspecified

Chapter 8 Functions of the skin and related structures

Functions of the skin (b810-b849)

b810 Protective functions of the skin
b820 Repair functions of the skin
b830 Other functions of the skin
b840 Sensation related to the skin
b849 Functions of the skin, other specified and unspecified

Functions of the hair and nails (b850-b869)

b850 Functions of hair
b860 Functions of nails
b869 Functions of the hair and nails, other specified and unspecified
b898 Functions of the skin and related structures, other specified
b899 Functions of the skin and related structures, unspecified

BODY STRUCTURES

Chapter 1 Structures of the nervous system
s110   Structure of brain
s120   Spinal cord and related structures
s130   Structure of meninges
s140   Structure of sympathetic nervous system
s150   Structure of parasympathetic nervous system
s198   Structure of the nervous system, other specified
s199   Structure of the nervous system, unspecified

Chapter 2 The eye, ear and related structures
s210   Structure of eye socket
s220   Structure of eyeball
s230   Structures around eye
s240   Structure of external ear
s250   Structure of middle ear
s260   Structure of inner ear
s298   Eye, ear and related structures, other specified
s299   Eye, ear and related structures, unspecified

Chapter 3 Structures involved in voice and speech
s310   Structure of nose
s320   Structure of mouth
s330   Structure of pharynx
s340   Structure of larynx
s398   Structures involved in voice and speech, other specified
s399   Structures involved in voice and speech, unspecified

Chapter 4 Structures of the cardiovascular, immunological and respiratory systems
s410   Structure of cardiovascular system
s420   Structure of immune system
s430   Structure of respiratory system
s498   Structures of the cardiovascular, immunological and respiratory systems, other specified
s499   Structures of the cardiovascular, immunological and respiratory systems, unspecified

Chapter 5 Structures related to the digestive, metabolic and endocrine systems
s510   Structure of salivary glands
s520   Structure of oesophagus
s530   Structure of stomach
s540   Structure of intestine
s550   Structure of pancreas
s560   Structure of liver

s570 Structure of gall bladder and ducts
s580 Structure of endocrine glands
s598 Structures related to the digestive, metabolic and endocrine systems, other specified
s599 Structures related to the digestive, metabolic and endocrine systems, unspecified

Chapter 6 Structures related to the genitourinary and reproductive systems

s610 Structure of urinary system
s620 Structure of pelvic floor
s630 Structure of reproductive system
s698 Structures related to the genitourinary and reproductive systems, other specified
s699 Structures related to the genitourinary and reproductive systems, unspecified

Chapter 7 Structures related to movement

s710 Structure of head and neck region
s720 Structure of shoulder region
s730 Structure of upper extremity
s740 Structure of pelvic region
s750 Structure of lower extremity
s760 Structure of trunk
s770 Additional musculoskeletal structures related to movement
s798 Structures related to movement, other specified
s799 Structures related to movement, unspecified

Chapter 8 Skin and related structures

s810 Structure of areas of skin
s820 Structure of skin glands
s830 Structure of nails
s840 Structure of hair
s898 Skin and related structures, other specified
s899 Skin and related structures, unspecifed

ACTIVITIES AND PARTICIPATION

Chapter 1 Learning and applying knowledge

Purposeful sensory experiences (d110-d129)

d110 Watching
d115 Listening
d120 Other purposeful sensing
d129 Purposeful sensory experiences, other specified and unspecified

Basic learning (d130-d159)

d130 Copying
d135 Rehearsing
d140 Learning to read
d145 Learning to write
d150 Learning to calculate
d155 Acquiring skills
d159 Basic learning, other specified and unspecified

Applying knowledge (d160-d179)

d160 Focusing attention
d163 Thinking
d166 Reading
d170 Writing
d172 Calculating
d175 Solving problems
d177 Making decisions
d179 Applying knowledge, other specified and unspecified
d198 Learning and applying knowledge, other specified
d199 Learning and applying knowledge, unspecified

Chapter 2 General tasks and demands

d210 Undertaking a single task
d220 Undertaking multiple tasks
d230 Carrying out daily routine
d240 Handling stress and other psychological demands
d298 General tasks and demands, other specified
d299 General tasks and demands, unspecified

Chapter 3 Communication

Communicating - receiving (d310-d329)

d310 Communicating with - receiving - spoken messages
d315 Communicating with - receiving - nonverbal messages
d320 Communicating with - receiving - formal sign language messages
d325 Communicating with - receiving - written messages
d329 Communicating - receiving, other specified and unspecified

Communicating - producing (d330-d349)

d330 Speaking
d335 Producing nonverbal messages
d340 Producing messages in formal sign language
d345 Writing messages
d349 Communication - producing, other specified and unspecified

Conversation and use of communication devices and techniques (d350-d369)

d350 Conversation
d355 Discussion
d360 Using communication devices and techniques
d369 Conversation and use of communication devices and techniques, other specified and unspecified
d398 Communication, other specified
d399 Communication, unspecified

Chapter 4 Mobility

Changing and maintaining body position (d410-d429)

d410 Changing basic body position
d415 Maintaining a body position
d420 Transferring oneself
d429 Changing and maintaining body position, other specified and unspecified

Carrying, moving and handling objects (d430-d449)

d430 Lifting and carrying objects
d435 Moving objects with lower extremities
d440 Fine hand use
d445 Hand and arm use
d449 Carrying, moving and handling objects, other specified and unspecified

Walking and moving (d450-d469)

d450 Walking
d455 Moving around
d460 Moving around in different locations
d465 Moving around using equipment
d469 Walking and moving, other specified and unspecified

Moving around using transportation (d470-d489)

d470 Using transportation
d475 Driving
d480 Riding animals for transportation
d489 Moving around using transportation, other specified and unspecified
d498 Mobility, other specified
d499 Mobility, unspecified

Chapter 5 Self-care

d510 Washing oneself
d520 Caring for body parts
d530 Toileting
d540 Dressing
d550 Eating
d560 Drinking
d570 Looking after one's health
d598 Self-care, other specified
d599 Self-care, unspecified

Chapter 6 Domestic life

Acquisition of necessities (d610-d629)
d610 Acquiring a place to live
d620 Acquisition of goods and services
d629 Acquisition of necessities, other specified and unspecified

Household tasks (d630-d649)
d630 Preparing meals
d640 Doing housework
d649 Household tasks, other specified and unspecified

Caring for household objects and assisting others (d650-d669)
d650 Caring for household objects
d660 Assisting others
d669 Caring for household objects and assisting others, other specified and
      unspecified
d698 Domestic life, other specified
d699 Domestic life, unspecified

Chapter 7 Interpersonal interactions and relationships

General interpersonal interactions (d710-d729)
d710 Basic interpersonal interactions
d720 Complex interpersonal interactions
d729 General interpersonal interactions, other specified and unspecified

Particular interpersonal relationships (d730-d779)
d730 Relating with strangers
d740 Formal relationships
d750 Informal social relationships
d760 Family relationships
d770 Intimate relationships
d779 Particular interpersonal relationships, other specified and unspecified
d798 Interpersonal interactions and relationships, other specified
d799 Interpersonal interactions and relationships, unspecified

Chapter 8 Major life areas

Education (d810-d839)
d810 Informal education
d815 Preschool education
d820 School education
d825 Vocational training
d830 Higher education
d839 Education, other specified and unspecified

Work and employment (d840-d859)
d840 Apprenticeship (work preparation)
d845 Acquiring, keeping and terminating a job
d850 Remunerative employment
d855 Non-remunerative employment
d859 Work and employment, other specified and unspecified

Economic life (d860-d879)
d860 Basic economic transactions
d865 Complex economic transactions
d870 Economic self-sufficiency
d879 Economic life, other specified and unspecified
d898 Major life areas, other specified
d899 Major life areas, unspecified

Chapter 9 Community, social and civic life
d910 Community life
d920 Recreation and leisure
d930 Religion and spirituality
d940 Human rights
d950 Political life and citizenship
d998 Community, social and civic life, other specified
d999 Community, social and civic life, unspecified

ENVIRONMENTAL FACTORS

Chapter 1 Products and technology
e110 Products or substances for personal consumption
e115 Products and technology for personal use in daily living
e120 Products and technology for personal indoor and outdoor mobility and transportation
e125 Products and technology for communication
e130 Products and technology for education
e135 Products and technology for employment
e140 Products and technology for culture, recreation and sport
e145 Products and technology for the practice of religion and spirituality
e150 Design, construction and building products and technology of buildings for public use
e155 Design, construction and building products and technology of buildings for private use
e160 Products and technology of land development
e165 Assets
e198 Products and technology, other specified
e199 Products and technology, unspecified

Chapter 2 Natural environment and human-made changes to environment
e210 Physical geography
e215 Population
e220 Flora and fauna
e225 Climate
e230 Natural events
e235 Human-caused events
e240 Light
e245 Time-related changes
e250 Sound
e255 Vibration
e260 Air quality
e298 Natural environment and human-made changes to environment, other specified
e299 Natural environment and human-made changes to environment, unspecified

Chapter 3 Support and relationships
e310 Immediate family
e315 Extended family
e320 Friends
e325 Acquaintances, peers colleagues, neighbours and community members
e330 People in positions of authority
e335 People in subordinate positions
e340 Personal care providers and personal assistants
e345 Strangers

e350 Domesticated animals
e355 Health professionals
e360 Health-related professionals
e398 Support and relationships, other specified
e399 Support and relationships, unspecified

Chapter 4 Attitudes

e410 Individual attitudes of immediate family members
e415 Individual attitudes of extended family members
e420 Individual attitudes of friends
e425 Individual attitudes of acquaintances, peers colleagues, neighbours and community members
e430 Individual attitudes of people in positions of authority
e435 Individual attitudes of people in subordinate positions
e440 Individual attitudes of personal care providers and personal assistants
e445 Individual attitudes of strangers
e450 Individual attitudes of health professionals
e455 Individual attitudes of health-related professionals
e460 Societal attitudes
e465 Social norms, practices and ideologies
e498 Attitudes, other specified
e499 Attitudes, unspecified

Chapter 5 Services, systems and policies

e510 Services, systems and policies for the production of consumer goods
e515 Architecture and construction services, systems and policies
e520 Open space planning services, systems and policies
e525 Housing services, systems and policies
e530 Utilities services, systems and policies
e535 Communication services, systems and policies
e540 Transportation services, systems and policies
e545 Civil protection services, systems and policies
e550 Legal services, systems and policies
e555 Associations and organizational services, systems and policies
e560 Media services, systems and policies
e565 Economic services, systems and policies
e570 Social security services, systems and policies
e575 General social support services, systems and policies
e580 Health services, systems and policies
e585 Education and training services, systems and policies
e590 Labour and employment services, systems and policies
e595 Political services, systems and policies
e598 Services, systems and policies, other specified
e599 Services, systems and policies, unspecified

ICF

Detailed classification with definitions

All categories within the classification with their definitions, inclusions and exclusions

BODY FUNCTIONS

Definitions: **Body functions** *are the physiological functions of body systems (including psychological functions).*

                        Impairments *are problems in body function or structure as a significant deviation or loss.*

Qualifier

Generic qualifier with the negative scale, used to indicate the extent or magnitude of an impairment:

xxx.0 NO impairment	(none, absent, negligible,…)	0-4 %
xxx.1 MILD impairment	(slight, low,…)	5-24 %
xxx.2 MODERATE impairment	(medium, fair,...)	25-49 %
xxx.3 SEVERE impairment	(high, extreme, …)	50-95 %
xxx.4 COMPLETE impairment	(total,…)	96-100 %
xxx.8 not specified		
xxx.9 not applicable		

Broad ranges of percentages are provided for those cases in which calibrated assessment instruments or other standards are available to quantify the impairment in body function. For example, when "no impairment" or "complete impairment" in body function is coded, this scaling may have margin of error of up to 5%. "Moderate impairment" is generally up to half of the scale of total impairment. The percentages are to be calibrated in different domains with reference to population standards as percentiles. For this quantification to be used in a uniform manner, assessment procedures need to be developed through research.

For a further explanation of coding conventions in ICF, refer to Annex 2.

Chapter 1
Mental functions

This chapter is about the functions of the brain: both global mental functions, such as consciousness, energy and drive, and specific mental functions, such as memory, language and calculation mental functions.

Global mental functions (b110-b139)

b110   **Consciousness functions**
General mental functions of the state of awareness and alertness, including the clarity and continuity of the wakeful state.

Inclusions: functions of the state, continuity and quality of consciousness; loss of consciousness, coma, vegetative states, fugues, trance states, possession states, drug-induced altered consciousness, delirium, stupor

Exclusions: orientation functions (b114); energy and drive functions (b130); sleep functions (b134)

   b1100   State of consciousness
   Mental functions that when altered produce states such as clouding of consciousness, stupor or coma.

   b1101   Continuity of consciousness
   Mental functions that produce sustained wakefulness, alertness and awareness and, when disrupted, may produce fugue, trance or other similar states.

   b1102   Quality of consciousness
   Mental functions that when altered effect changes in the character of wakeful, alert and aware sentience, such as drug-induced altered states or delirium.

   b1108   Consciousness functions, other specified

   b1109   Consciousness functions, unspecified

b114   **Orientation functions**
General mental functions of knowing and ascertaining one's relation to self, to others, to time and to one's surroundings.

Inclusions: functions of orientation to time, place and person; orientation to self and others; disorientation to time, place and person

Exclusions: consciousness functions (b110); attention functions (b140); memory functions (b144)

b 1140   Orientation to time
Mental functions that produce awareness of day, date, month and year.

b 1141   Orientation to place
Mental functions that produce awareness of one's location, such as one's immediate surroundings, one's town or country.

b 1142   Orientation to person
Mental functions that produce awareness of one's own identity and of individuals in the immediate environment.

    b 11420   Orientation to self
    Mental functions that produce awareness of one's own identity.

    b 11421   Orientation to others
    Mental functions that produce awareness of the identity of other individuals in one's immediate environment .

    b 11428   Orientation to person, other specified

    b 11429   Orientation to person, unspecified

b 1148   Orientation functions, other specified

b 1149   Orientation functions, unspecified

b117   **Intellectual functions**
General mental functions, required to understand and constructively integrate the various mental functions, including all cognitive functions and their development over the life span.

Inclusions: functions of intellectual growth; intellectual retardation, mental retardation, dementia

Exclusions: memory functions (b144); thought functions (b160); higher-level cognitive functions (b164)

b122   **Global psychosocial functions**
General mental functions, as they develop over the life span, required to understand and constructively integrate the mental functions that lead to the formation of the interpersonal skills needed to establish reciprocal social interactions, in terms of both meaning and purpose.

Inclusion: such as in autism

b 126 **Temperament and personality functions**
General mental functions of constitutional disposition of the individual to react in a particular way to situations, including the set of mental characteristics that makes the individual distinct from others.

Inclusions: functions of extraversion, introversion, agreeableness, conscientiousness, psychic and emotional stability, and openness to experience; optimism; novelty seeking; confidence; trustworthiness

Exclusions: intellectual functions (b117); energy and drive functions (b130); psychomotor functions (b147); emotional functions (b152)

> **b 1260** **Extraversion**
> Mental functions that produce a personal disposition that is outgoing, sociable and demonstrative, as contrasted to being shy, restricted and inhibited.

> **b 1261** **Agreeableness**
> Mental functions that produce a personal disposition that is cooperative, amicable, and accommodating, as contrasted to being unfriendly, oppositional and defiant.

> **b 1262** **Conscientiousness**
> Mental functions that produce personal dispositions such as in being hard-working, methodical and scrupulous, as contrasted to mental functions producing dispositions such as in being lazy, unreliable and irresponsible.

> **b 1263** **Psychic stability**
> Mental functions that produce a personal disposition that is even-tempered, calm and composed, as contrasted to being irritable, worried, erratic and moody.

> **b 1264** **Openness to experience**
> Mental functions that produce a personal disposition that is curious, imaginative, inquisitive and experience-seeking, as contrasted to being stagnant, inattentive and emotionally inexpressive.

> **b 1265** **Optimism**
> Mental functions that produce a personal disposition that is cheerful, buoyant and hopeful, as contrasted to being downhearted, gloomy and despairing.

b 1266   Confidence
Mental functions that produce a personal disposition that is
self-assured, bold and assertive, as contrasted to being timid,
insecure and self-effacing.

b 1267   Trustworthiness
Mental functions that produce a personal disposition that is
dependable and principled, as contrasted to being deceitful
and antisocial.

b 1268   Temperament and personality functions, other specified

b 1269   Temperament and personality functions, unspecified

b 130   Energy and drive functions
General mental functions of physiological and psychological
mechanisms that cause the individual to move towards satisfying
specific needs and general goals in a persistent manner.

*Inclusions: functions of energy level, motivation, appetite, craving
(including craving for substances that can be abused), and impulse control*

*Exclusions: consciousness functions (b110); temperament and personality
functions (b126); sleep functions (b134); psychomotor functions (b147);
emotional functions (b152)*

b 1300   Energy level
Mental functions that produce vigour and stamina.

b 1301   Motivation
Mental functions that produce the incentive to act; the
conscious or unconscious driving force for action.

b 1302   Appetite
Mental functions that produce a natural longing or desire,
especially the natural and recurring desire for food and drink.

b 1303   Craving
Mental functions that produce the urge to consume substances,
including substances that can be abused.

b 1304   Impulse control
Mental functions that regulate and resist sudden intense urges
to do something.

b 1308   Energy and drive functions, other specified

b 1309   Energy and drive functions, unspecified

b 134   Sleep functions
General mental functions of periodic, reversible and selective physical and mental disengagement from one's immediate environment accompanied by characteristic physiological changes.

Inclusions: functions of amount of sleeping, and onset, maintenance and quality of sleep; functions involving the sleep cycle, such as in insomnia, hypersomnia and narcolepsy

Exclusions: consciousness functions (b110); energy and drive functions (b130); attention functions (b140); psychomotor functions (b147)

b 1340   Amount of sleep
Mental functions involved in the time spent in the state of sleep in the diurnal cycle or circadian rhythm.

b 1341   Onset of sleep
Mental functions that produce the transition between wakefulness and sleep.

b 1342   Maintenance of sleep
Mental functions that sustain the state of being asleep.

b 1343   Quality of sleep
Mental functions that produce the natural sleep leading to optimal physical and mental rest and relaxation.

b 1344   Functions involving the sleep cycle
Mental functions that produce rapid eye movement (REM) sleep (associated with dreaming) and non-rapid eye movement sleep (NREM) (characterized by the traditional concept of sleep as a time of decreased physiological and psychological activity).

b 1348   Sleep functions, other specified

b 1349   Sleep functions, unspecified

b 139   Global mental functions, other specified and unspecified

Specific mental functions (b140-b189)

b140 **Attention functions**
Specific mental functions of focusing on an external stimulus or internal experience for the required period of time.

Inclusions: functions of sustaining attention, shifting attention, dividing attention, sharing attention; concentration; distractibility

Exclusions: consciousness functions (b110); energy and drive functions (b130); sleep functions (b134); memory functions (b144); psychomotor functions (b147); perceptual functions (b156)

b1400 **Sustaining attention**
Mental functions that produce concentration for the period of time required.

b1401 **Shifting attention**
Mental functions that permit refocusing concentration from one stimulus to another.

b1402 **Dividing attention**
Mental functions that permit focusing on two or more stimuli at the same time.

b1403 **Sharing attention**
Mental functions that permit focusing on the same stimulus by two or more people, such as a child and a caregiver both focusing on a toy.

b1408 **Attention functions, other specified**

b1409 **Attention functions, unspecified**

b144 **Memory functions**
Specific mental functions of registering and storing information and retrieving it as needed.

Inclusions: functions of short-term and long-term memory, immediate, recent and remote memory; memory span; retrieval of memory; remembering; functions used in recalling and learning, such as in nominal, selective and dissociative amnesia

Exclusions: consciousness functions (b110); orientation functions (b114); intellectual functions (b117); attention functions (b140); perceptual functions (b156); thought functions (b160); higher-level cognitive functions (b164); mental functions of language (b167); calculation functions (b172)

b1440 Short-term memory
Mental functions that produce a temporary, disruptable memory store of around 30 seconds duration from which information is lost if not consolidated into long-term memory.

b1441 Long-term memory
Mental functions that produce a memory system permitting the long-term storage of information from short-term memory and both autobiographical memory for past events and semantic memory for language and facts.

b1442 Retrieval of memory
Specific mental functions of recalling information stored in long-term memory and bringing it into awareness.

b1448 Memory functions, other specified

b1449 Memory functions, unspecified

b147 Psychomotor functions
Specific mental functions of control over both motor and psychological events at the body level.

Inclusions: functions of psychomotor control, such as psychomotor retardation, excitement and agitation, posturing, catatonia, negativism, ambitendency, echopraxia and echolalia; quality of psychomotor function

Exclusions: consciousness functions (b110); orientation functions (b114); intellectual functions (b117); energy and drive functions (b130); attention functions (b140); mental functions of language (b167); mental functions of sequencing complex movements (b176)

b1470 Psychomotor control
Mental functions that regulate the speed of behaviour or response time that involves both motor and psychological components, such as in disruption of control producing psychomotor retardation (moving and speaking slowly; decrease in gesturing and spontaneity) or psychomotor excitement (excessive behavioural and cognitive activity, usually nonproductive and often in response to inner tension as in toe-tapping, hand-wringing, agitation, or restlessness.)

b1471 Quality of psychomotor functions
Mental functions that produce nonverbal behaviour in the proper sequence and character of its subcomponents, such as hand and eye coordination, or gait.

b1478 Psychomotor functions, other specified

b 1479   Psychomotor functions, unspecified

b 152   **Emotional functions**
Specific mental functions related to the feeling and affective components
of the processes of the mind.

*Inclusions: functions of appropriateness of emotion, regulation and range
of emotion; affect; sadness, happiness, love, fear, anger, hate, tension,
anxiety, joy, sorrow; lability of emotion; flattening of affect*

*Exclusions: temperament and personality functions (b126); energy and
drive functions (b130)*

b 1520   Appropriateness of emotion
Mental functions that produce congruence of feeling or affect
with the situation, such as happiness at receiving good news.

b 1521   Regulation of emotion
Mental functions that control the experience and display of
affect.

b 1522   Range of emotion
Mental functions that produce the spectrum of experience of
arousal of affect or feelings such as love, hate, anxiousness,
sorrow, joy, fear and anger.

b 1528   Emotional functions, other specified

b 1529   Emotional functions, unspecified

b 156   **Perceptual functions**
Specific mental functions of recognizing and interpreting sensory
stimuli.

*Inclusions: functions of auditory, visual, olfactory, gustatory, tactile and
visuospatial perception, such as hallucination or illusion*

*Exclusions: consciousness functions (b110); orientation functions (b114);
attention functions (b140); memory functions (b144); mental functions of
language (b167); seeing and related functions (b210-b229); hearing and
vestibular functions (b230-b249); additional sensory functions (b250-
b279)*

b 1560   Auditory perception
Mental functions involved in discriminating sounds, tones,
pitches and other acoustic stimuli.

b 1561   Visual perception
Mental functions involved in discriminating shape, size, colour and other ocular stimuli.

b 1562   Olfactory perception
Mental functions involved in distinguishing differences in smells.

b 1563   Gustatory perception
Mental functions involved in distinguishing differences in tastes, such as sweet, sour, salty and bitter stimuli, detected by the tongue.

b 1564   Tactile perception
Mental functions involved in distinguishing differences in texture, such as rough or smooth stimuli, detected by touch.

b 1565   Visuospatial perception
Mental function involved in distinguishing by sight the relative position of objects in the environment or in relation to oneself.

b 1568   Perceptual functions, other specified

b 1569   Perceptual functions, unspecified

b160   Thought functions
Specific mental functions related to the ideational component of the mind.

Inclusions: functions of pace, form, control and content of thought; goal-directed thought functions, non-goal directed thought functions; logical thought functions, such as pressure of thought, flight of ideas, thought block, incoherence of thought, tangentiality, circumstantiality, delusions, obsessions and compulsions

Exclusions: intellectual functions (b117); memory functions (b144); psychomotor functions (b147); perceptual functions (b156); higher-level cognitive functions (b164); mental functions of language (b167); calculation functions (b172)

b 1600   Pace of thought
Mental functions that govern speed of the thinking process.

b 1601   Form of thought
Mental functions that organize the thinking process as to its coherence and logic.

Inclusions: impairments of ideational perseveration, tangentiality and circumstantiality

b 1602   Content of thought
Mental functions consisting of the ideas that are present in the thinking process and what is being conceptualized.

Inclusions: impairments of delusions, overvalued ideas and somatization

b 1603   Control of thought
Mental functions that provide volitional control of thinking and are recognized as such by the person.

Inclusions: impairments of rumination, obsession, thought broadcast and thought insertion

b 1608   Thought functions, other specified

b 1609   Thought functions, unspecified

b 164   Higher-level cognitive functions
Specific mental functions especially dependent on the frontal lobes of the brain, including complex goal-directed behaviours such as decision-making, abstract thinking, planning and carrying out plans, mental flexibility, and deciding which behaviours are appropriate under what circumstances; often called executive functions.

Inclusions: functions of abstraction and organization of ideas; time management, insight and judgement; concept formation, categorization and cognitive flexibility

Exclusions: memory functions (b144); thought functions (b160); mental functions of language (b167); calculation functions (b172)

b 1640   Abstraction
Mental functions of creating general ideas, qualities or characteristics out of, and distinct from, concrete realities, specific objects or actual instances.

b 1641   Organization and planning
Mental functions of coordinating parts into a whole, of systematizing; the mental function involved in developing a method of proceeding or acting.

b 1642   Time management
Mental functions of ordering events in chronological sequence, allocating amounts of time to events and activities.

b 1643   Cognitive flexibility
Mental functions of changing strategies, or shifting mental sets, especially as involved in problem-solving.

b 1644   Insight
Mental functions of awareness and understanding of oneself and one's behaviour.

b 1645   Judgement
Mental functions involved in discriminating between and evaluating different options, such as those involved in forming an opinion.

b 1646   Problem-solving
Mental functions of identifying, analysing and integrating incongruent or conflicting information into a solution.

b 1648   Higher-level cognitive functions, other specified

b 1649   Higher-level cognitive functions, unspecified

b 167   Mental functions of language
Specific mental functions of recognizing and using signs, symbols and other components of a language.

Inclusions: functions of reception and decryption of spoken, written or other forms of language such as sign language; functions of expression of spoken, written or other forms of language; integrative language functions, spoken and written, such as involved in receptive, expressive, Broca's, Wernicke's and conduction aphasia

Exclusions: attention functions (b140); memory functions (b144); perceptual functions (b156); thought functions (b160); higher-level cognitive functions (b164); calculation functions (b172); mental functions of complex movements (b176); Chapter 2 Sensory Functions and Pain; Chapter 3 Voice and Speech Functions

b 1670   Reception of language
Specific mental functions of decoding messages in spoken, written or other forms, such as sign language, to obtain their meaning.

b 16700 Reception of spoken language
Mental functions of decoding spoken messages to
obtain their meaning.

b 16701 Reception of written language
Mental functions of decoding written messages to
obtain their meaning.

b 16702 Reception of sign language
Mental functions of decoding messages in languages
that use signs made by hands and other movements,
in order to obtain their meaning.

b 16708 Reception of language, other specified

b 16709 Reception of language, unspecified

b 1671 Expression of language
Specific mental functions necessary to produce meaningful
messages in spoken, written, signed or other forms of language.

b 16710 Expression of spoken language
Mental functions necessary to produce meaningful
spoken messages.

b 16711 Expression of written language
Mental functions necessary to produce meaningful
written messages.

b 16712 Expression of sign language
Mental functions necessary to produce meaningful
messages in languages that use signs made by hands
and other movements.

b 16718 Expression of language, other specified

b 16719 Expression of language, unspecified

b 1672 Integrative language functions
Mental functions that organize semantic and symbolic
meaning, grammatical structure and ideas for the production
of messages in spoken, written or other forms of language.

b 1678 Mental functions of language, other specified

b 1679 Mental functions of language, unspecified

b172   Calculation functions
Specific mental functions of determination, approximation and manipulation of mathematical symbols and processes.

Inclusions: functions of addition, subtraction, and other simple mathematical calculations; functions of complex mathematical operations

Exclusions: attention functions (b140); memory functions (b144); thought functions (b160); higher-level cognitive functions (b164); mental functions of language (b167)

b1720   Simple calculation
Mental functions of computing with numbers, such as addition, subtraction, multiplication and division.

b1721   Complex calculation
Mental functions of translating word problems into arithmetic procedures, translating mathematical formulas into arithmetic procedures, and other complex manipulations involving numbers.

b1728   Calculation functions, other specified

b1729   Calculation functions, unspecified

b176   Mental function of sequencing complex movements
Specific mental functions of sequencing and coordinating complex, purposeful movements.

Inclusions: impairments such as in ideation, ideomotor, dressing, oculomotor and speech apraxia

Exclusions: psychomotor functions (b147); higher-level cognitive functions (b164); Chapter 7 Neuromusculoskeletal and Movement-Related Functions

b180   Experience of self and time functions
Specific mental functions related to the awareness of one's identity, one's body, one's position in the reality of one's environment and of time.

Inclusions: functions of experience of self, body image and time

b1800   Experience of self
Specific mental functions of being aware of one's own identity and one's position in the reality of the environment around oneself.

Inclusion: impairments such as depersonalization and derealization

60

b 1801   Body image
Specific mental functions related to the representation and
awareness of one's body.

*Inclusion: impairments such as phantom limb and feeling too fat
or too thin*

b 1802   Experience of time
Specific mental functions of the subjective experiences related
to the length and passage of time.

Inclusion: impairments such as jamais vu and déjà vu

b 1808   Experience of self and time functions, other specified

b 1809   Experience of self and time functions, unspecified

b 189   Specific mental functions, other specified and unspecified

b 198   Mental functions, other specified

b 199   Mental functions, unspecified

Chapter 2
Sensory functions and pain

This chapter is about the functions of the senses, seeing, hearing, tasting and so on, as well as the sensation of pain.

Seeing and related functions (b210-b229)

b210 **Seeing functions**
Sensory functions relating to sensing the presence of light and sensing the form, size, shape and colour of the visual stimuli.

Inclusions: visual acuity functions; visual field functions; quality of vision; functions of sensing light and colour, visual acuity of distant and near vision, monocular and binocular vision; visual picture quality; impairments such as myopia, hypermetropia, astigmatism, hemianopia, colour-blindness, tunnel vision, central and peripheral scotoma, diplopia, night blindness and impaired adaptability to light

Exclusion: perceptual functions (b156)

b2100 **Visual acuity functions**
Seeing functions of sensing form and contour, both binocular and monocular, for both distant and near vision.

b21000 **Binocular acuity of distant vision**
Seeing functions of sensing size, form and contour, using both eyes, for objects distant from the eye.

b21001 **Monocular acuity of distant vision**
Seeing functions of sensing size, form and contour, using either right or left eye alone, for objects distant from the eye.

b21002 **Binocular acuity of near vision**
Seeing functions of sensing size, form and contour, using both eyes, for objects close to the eye.

b21003 **Monocular acuity of near vision**
Seeing functions of sensing size, form and contour, using either right or left eye alone, for objects close to the eye.

b21008 **Visual acuity functions, other specified**

b21009 **Visual acuity functions, unspecified**

b 2101 Visual field functions
Seeing functions related to the entire area that can be seen with fixation of gaze.

Inclusions: impairments such as in scotoma, tunnel vision, anopsia

b 2102 Quality of vision
Seeing functions involving light sensitivity, colour vision, contrast sensitivity and the overall quality of the picture.

b 21020 Light sensitivity
Seeing functions of sensing a minimum amount of light (light minimum), and the minimum difference in intensity (light difference.)

Inclusions: functions of dark adaptation; impairments such as night blindness (hyposensitivity to light) and photophobia (hypersensitivity to light)

b 21021 Colour vision
Seeing functions of differentiating and matching colours.

b 21022 Contrast sensitivity
Seeing functions of separating figure from ground, involving the minimum amount of luminance required.

b 21023 Visual picture quality
Seeing functions involving the quality of the picture.

Inclusions: impairments such as in seeing stray lights, affected picture quality (floaters or webbing), picture distortion, and seeing stars or flashes

b 21028 Quality of vision, other specified

b 21029 Quality of vision, unspecified

b 2108 Seeing functions, other specified

b 2109 Seeing functions, unspecified

b215 Functions of structures adjoining the eye
Functions of structures in and around the eye that facilitate seeing functions.

Inclusions: functions of internal muscles of the eye, eyelid, external muscles of the eye, including voluntary and tracking movements and fixation of the eye, lachrymal glands, accommodation, pupillary reflex; impairments such as in nystagmus, xerophthalmia and ptosis

Exclusions: seeing functions (b210); Chapter 7 Neuromusculoskeletal and Movement-related Functions

b 2150 **Functions of internal muscles of the eye**
Functions of the muscles inside the eye, such as the iris, that adjust the shape and size of the pupil and lens of the eye.

Inclusions: functions of accommodation; pupillary reflex

b 2151 **Functions of the eyelid**
Functions of the eyelid, such as the protective reflex.

b 2152 **Functions of external muscles of the eye**
Functions of the muscles that are used to look in different directions, to follow an object as it moves across the visual field, to produce saccadic jumps to catch up with a moving target, and to fix the eye.

Inclusions: nystagmus; cooperation of both eyes

b 2153 **Functions of lachrymal glands**
Functions of the tear glands and ducts.

b 2158 **Functions of structures adjoining the eye, other specified**

b 2159 **Functions of structures adjoining the eye, unspecified**

b 220 Sensations associated with the eye and adjoining structures
Sensations of tired, dry and itching eye and related feelings.

Inclusions: feelings of pressure behind the eye, of something in the eye, eye strain, burning in the eye; eye irritation

Exclusion: sensation of pain (b280)

b 229 Seeing and related functions, other specified and unspecified

Hearing and vestibular functions (b230-b249)

b230   Hearing functions
Sensory functions relating to sensing the presence of sounds and discriminating the location, pitch, loudness and quality of sounds.

Inclusions: functions of hearing, auditory discrimination, localization of sound source, lateralization of sound, speech discrimination; impairments such as deafness, hearing impairment and hearing loss

Exclusions: perceptual functions (b156) and mental functions of language (b167)

   b2300   Sound detection
Sensory functions relating to sensing the presence of sounds.

   b2301   Sound discrimination
Sensory functions relating to sensing the presence of sound involving the differentiation of ground and binaural synthesis, separation and blending.

   b2302   Localisation of sound source
Sensory functions relating to determining the location of the source of sound.

   b2303   Lateralization of sound
Sensory functions relating to determining whether the sound is coming from the right or left side.

   b2304   Speech discrimination
Sensory functions relating to determining spoken language and distinguishing it from other sounds.

   b2308   Hearing functions, other specified

   b2309   Hearing functions, unspecified

b235   Vestibular functions
Sensory functions of the inner ear related to position, balance and movement.

Inclusions: functions of position and positional sense; functions of balance of the body and movement

Exclusion: sensation associated with hearing and vestibular functions (b240)

b 2350   **Vestibular function of position**
Sensory functions of the inner ear related to determining the position of the body.

b 2351   **Vestibular function of balance**
Sensory functions of the inner ear related to determining the balance of the body.

b 2352   **Vestibular function of determination of movement**
Sensory functions of the inner ear related to determining movement of the body, including its direction and speed.

b 2358   **Vestibular functions, other specified**

b 2359   **Vestibular functions, unspecified**

b 240   **Sensations associated with hearing and vestibular function**
Sensations of dizziness, falling, tinnitus and vertigo.

Inclusions: sensations of ringing in ears, irritation in ear, aural pressure, nausea associated with dizziness or vertigo

Exclusions: vestibular functions (b235); sensation of pain (b280)

b 2400   **Ringing in ears or tinnitus**
Sensation of low-pitched rushing, hissing or ringing in the ear.

b 2401   **Dizziness**
Sensation of motion involving either oneself or one's environment; sensation of rotating, swaying or tilting.

b 2402   **Sensation of falling**
Sensation of losing one's grip and falling.

b 2403   **Nausea associated with dizziness or vertigo**
Sensation of wanting to vomit that arises from dizziness or vertigo.

b 2404   **Irritation in the ear**
Sensation of itching or other similar sensations in the ear.

b 2405   **Aural pressure**
Sensation of pressure in the ear.

b 2408   **Sensations associated with hearing and vestibular function, other specified**

      b 2409   Sensations associated with hearing and vestibular function, unspecified

b 249   Hearing and vestibular functions, other specified and unspecified

Additional sensory functions (b250-b279)

b 250   Taste function
Sensory functions of sensing qualities of bitterness, sweetness, sourness and saltiness.

Inclusions: gustatory functions; impairments such as ageusia and hypogeusia

b 255   Smell function
Sensory functions of sensing odours and smells.

Inclusions: olfactory functions; impairments such as anosmia or hyposmia

b 260   Proprioceptive function
Sensory functions of sensing the relative position of body parts.

Inclusions: functions of statesthesia and kinaesthesia

Exclusions: vestibular functions (b235); sensations related to muscles and movement functions (b780)

b 265   Touch function
Sensory functions of sensing surfaces and their texture or quality.

Inclusions: functions of touching, feeling of touch; impairments such as numbness, anaesthesia, tingling, paraesthesia and hyperaesthesia

Exclusions: sensory functions related to temperature and other stimuli (b270)

b 270   Sensory functions related to temperature and other stimuli
Sensory functions of sensing temperature, vibration, pressure and noxious stimulus.

Inclusions: functions of being sensitive to temperature, vibration, shaking or oscillation, superficial pressure, deep pressure, burning sensation or a noxious stimulus

Exclusions: touch functions (b265); sensation of pain (b280)

      b 2700   Sensitivity to temperature
               Sensory functions of sensing cold and heat.

b 2701 **Sensitivity to vibration**
Sensory functions of sensing shaking or oscillation.

b 2702 **Sensitivity to pressure**
Sensory functions of sensing pressure against or on the skin.

Inclusions: impairments such as sensitivity to touch, numbness, hypaesthesia, hyperaesthesia, paraesthesia and tingling

b 2703 **Sensitivity to a noxious stimulus**
Sensory functions of sensing painful or uncomfortable sensations.

Inclusions: impairments such as hypalgesia, hyperpathia, allodynia, analgesia and anaesthesia dolorosa

b 2708 **Sensory functions related to temperature and other stimuli, other specified**

b 2709 **Sensory functions related to temperature and other stimuli, unspecified**

b 279 Additional sensory functions, other specified and unspecified

Pain (b280-b289)

b 280 Sensation of pain
Sensation of unpleasant feeling indicating potential or actual damage to some body structure.

Inclusions: sensations of generalized or localized pain, in one or more body part, pain in a dermatome, stabbing pain, burning pain, dull pain, aching pain; impairments such as myalgia, analgesia and hyperalgesia

b 2800 **Generalized pain**
Sensation of unpleasant feeling indicating potential or actual damage to some body structure felt all over, or throughout the body.

b 2801 **Pain in body part**
Sensation of unpleasant feeling indicating potential or actual damage to some body structure felt in a specific part, or parts, of the body.

b 28010 Pain in head and neck
Sensation of unpleasant feeling indicating potential or actual damage to some body structure felt in the head and neck.

b 28011 Pain in chest
Sensation of unpleasant feeling indicating potential or actual damage to some body structure felt in the chest.

b 28012 Pain in stomach or abdomen
Sensation of unpleasant feeling indicating potential or actual damage to some body structure felt in the stomach or abdomen.

Inclusion: pain in the pelvic region

b 28013 Pain in back
Sensation of unpleasant feeling indicating potential or actual damage to some body structure felt in the back.

Inclusions: pain in the trunk; low backache

b 28014 Pain in upper limb
Sensation of unpleasant feeling indicating potential or actual damage to some body structure felt in either one or both upper limbs, including hands.

b 28015 Pain in lower limb
Sensation of unpleasant feeling indicating potential or actual damage to some body structure felt in either one or both lower limbs, including feet.

b 28016 Pain in joints
Sensation of unpleasant feeling indicating potential or actual damage to some body structure felt in one or more joints, including small and big joints.

Inclusions: pain in the hip; pain in the shoulder

b 28018 Pain in body part, other specified

b 28019 Pain in body part, unspecified

b 2802 Pain in multiple body parts
Unpleasant sensation indicating potential or actual damage to some body structure located in several body parts.

b 2803   **Radiating pain in a dermatome**
Unpleasant sensation indicating potential or actual damage to
some body structure located in areas of skin served by the same
nerve root.

b 2804   **Radiating pain in a segment or region**
Unpleasant sensation indicating potential or actual damage to
some body structure located in areas of skin in different body
parts not served by the same nerve root.

b 289   Sensation of pain, other specified and unspecified

b 298   Sensory functions and pain, other specified

b 299   Sensory functions and pain, unspecified

Chapter 3
Voice and speech functions

This chapter is about the functions of producing sounds and speech.

b310   **Voice functions**
Functions of the production of various sounds by the passage of air through the larynx.

Inclusions: functions of production and quality of voice; functions of phonation, pitch, loudness and other qualities of voice; impairments such as aphonia, dysphonia, hoarseness, hypernasality and hyponasality

Exclusions: mental functions of language (b167); articulation functions (b320)

b 3100   **Production of voice**
Functions of the production of sound made through coordination of the larynx and surrounding muscles with the respiratory system.

Inclusions: functions of phonation, loudness; impairment of aphonia

b 3101   **Quality of voice**
Functions of the production of characteristics of voice including pitch, resonance and other features.

Inclusions: functions of high or low pitch; impairments such as hypernasality, hyponasality, dysphonia, hoarseness or harshness

b 3108   **Voice functions, other specified**

b 3109   **Voice functions, unspecified**

b320   **Articulation functions**
Functions of the production of speech sounds.

Inclusions: functions of enunciation, articulation of phonemes; spastic, ataxic, flaccid dysarthria; anarthria

Exclusions: mental functions of language (b167); voice functions (b310)

b 330 **Fluency and rhythm of speech functions**
Functions of the production of flow and tempo of speech.

*Inclusions: functions of fluency, rhythm, speed and melody of speech;
prosody and intonation; impairments such as stuttering, stammering,
cluttering, bradylalia and tachylalia*

*Exclusions: mental functions of language (b167); voice functions (b310);
articulation functions (b320)*

b 3300 **Fluency of speech**
Functions of the production of smooth, uninterrupted flow of
speech.

*Inclusions: functions of smooth connection of speech;
impairments such as stuttering, stammering, cluttering,
dysfluency, repetition of sounds, words or parts of words and
irregular breaks in speech*

b 3301 **Rhythm of speech**
Functions of the modulated, tempo and stress patterns in
speech.

*Inclusions: impairments such as stereotypic or repetitive speech
cadence*

b 3302 **Speed of speech**
Functions of the rate of speech production.

Inclusions: impairments such as bradylalia and tachylalia

b 3303 **Melody of speech**
Functions of modulation of pitch patterns in speech.

*Inclusions: prosody of speech, intonation, melody of speech;
impairments such as monotone speech*

b 3308 **Fluency and rhythm of speech functions, other specified**

b 3309 **Fluency and rhythm of speech functions, unspecified**

b 340 **Alternative vocalization functions**
Functions of the production of other manners of vocalization.

*Inclusions: functions of the production of notes and range of sounds, such
as in singing, chanting, babbling and humming; crying aloud and
screaming*

*Exclusions: mental functions of language (b167); voice functions (b310);
articulation functions (b320); fluency and rhythm of speech functions
(b330)*

b 3400   Production of notes
Functions of production of musical vocal sounds.

Inclusions: sustaining, modulating and terminating production of single or connected vocalizations with variation in pitch such as in singing, humming and chanting

b 3401   Making a range of sounds
Functions of production of a variety of vocalizations.

Inclusion: functions of babbling in children

b 3408   Alternative vocalization functions, other specified

b 3409   Alternative vocalization functions, unspecified

b 398   Voice and speech functions, other specified

b 399   Voice and speech functions, unspecified

Chapter 4

Functions of the cardiovascular, haematological, immunological and respiratory systems

This chapter is about the functions involved in the cardiovascular system (functions of the heart and blood vessels), the haematological and immunological systems (functions of blood production and immunity), and the respiratory system (functions of respiration and exercise tolerance).

Functions of the cardiovascular system (b410-b429)

b410 **Heart functions**

Functions of pumping the blood in adequate or required amounts and pressure throughout the body.

Inclusions: functions of heart rate, rhythm and output; contraction force of ventricular muscles; functions of heart valves; pumping the blood through the pulmonary circuit; dynamics of circulation to the heart; impairments such as tachycardia, bradycardia and irregular heart beatand as in heart failure, cardiomyopathy, myocarditis,and coronary insufficiency

Exclusions: blood vessel functions (b415); blood pressure functions (b420); exercise tolerance functions (b455)

b 4100 **Heart rate**

Functions related to the number of times the heart contracts every minute.

Inclusions: impairments such as rates that are too fast (tachycardia) or too slow (bradycardia)

b 4101 **Heart rhythm**

Functions related to the regularity of the beating of the heart.

Inclusions: impairments such as arrhythmias

b 4102 **Contraction force of ventricular muscles**

Functions related to the amount of blood pumped by the ventricular muscles during every beat.

Inclusions: impairments such as diminished cardiac output

b 4103   **Blood supply to the heart**
Functions related to the volume of blood available to the heart muscle.

Inclusion: impairments such as coronary ischaemia

b 4108   **Heart functions, other specified**

b 4109   **Heart functions, unspecified**

b415   **Blood vessel functions**
Functions of transporting blood throughout the body.

Inclusions: functions of arteries, capillaries and veins; vasomotor function; functions of pulmonary arteries, capillaries and veins; functions of valves of veins; impairments such as in blockage or constriction of arteries; atherosclerosis, arteriosclerosis, thromboembolism and varicose veins

Exclusions: heart functions (b410); blood pressure functions (b420); haematological system functions (b430); exercise tolerance functions (b455)

b 4150   **Functions of arteries**
functions related to blood flow in the arteries

Inclusions: impairments such as arterial dilation; arterial constriction such as in intermittent claudication

b 4151   **Functions of capillaries**
Functions related to blood flow in the capillaries.

b 4152   **Functions of veins**
Functions related to blood flow in the veins, and the functions of valves of veins.

Inclusions: impairments such as venous dilation; venous constriction; insufficient closing of valves as in varicose veins

b 4158   **Blood vessel functions, other specified**

b 4159   **Blood vessel functions, unspecified**

b420 **Blood pressure functions**
Functions of maintaining the pressure of blood within the arteries.

Inclusions: functions of maintenance of blood pressure; increased and decreased blood pressure; impairments such as in hypotension, hypertension and postural hypotension

Exclusions: heart functions (b410); blood vessel functions (b415); exercise tolerance functions (b455)

> **b4200** **Increased blood pressure**
> Functions related to a rise in systolic or diastolic blood pressure above normal for the age.

> **b4201** **Decreased blood pressure**
> Functions related to a fall in systolic or diastolic blood pressure below normal for the age.

> **b4202** **Maintenance of blood pressure**
> Functions related to maintaining an appropriate blood pressure in response to changes in the body.

> **b4208** **Blood pressure functions, other specified**

> **b4209** **Blood pressure functions, unspecified**

b429 Functions of the cardiovascular system, other specified and unspecified

Functions of the haematological and immunological systems (b430-b439)

b430 **Haematological system functions**
Functions of blood production, oxygen and metabolite carriage, and clotting.

Inclusions: functions of the production of blood and bone marrow; oxygen-carrying functions of blood; blood-related functions of spleen; metabolite-carrying functions of blood; clotting; impairments such as anaemia, haemophilia and other clotting dysfunctions

Exclusions: functions of the cardiovascular system (b410-b429); immunological system functions (b435); exercise tolerance functions (b455)

> **b4300** **Production of blood**
> Functions related to the production of blood and all its constituents.

b 4301   Oxygen-carrying functions of the blood
Functions related to the blood's capacity to carry oxygen
throughout the body.

b 4302   Metabolite-carrying functions of the blood
Functions related to the blood's capacity to carry metabolites
throughout the body.

b 4303   Clotting functions
Functions related to the coagulation of blood, such as at a site
of injury.

b 4308   Haematological system functions, other specified

b 4309   Haematological system functions, unspecified

b435   **Immunological system functions**
Functions of the body related to protection against foreign substances,
including infections, by specific and non-specific immune responses.

*Inclusions: immune response (specific and non-specific); hypersensitivity
reactions; functions of lymphatic vessels and nodes; functions of cell-
mediated immunity, antibody-mediated immunity; response to
immunization; impairments such as in autoimmunity, allergic reactions,
lymphadenitis and lymphoedema*

Exclusion: haematological system functions (b430)

b 4350   Immune response
Functions of the body's response of sensitization to foreign
substances, including infections.

b 43500   Specific immune response
Functions of the body's response of sensitization to a
specific foreign substance.

b 43501   Non-specific immune response
Functions of the body's general response of
sensitization to foreign substances, including
infections.

b 43508   Immune response, other specified

b 43509   Immune response, unspecified

b 4351   **Hypersensitivity reactions**
Functions of the body's response of increased sensitization to
foreign substances, such as in sensitivities to different antigens.

Inclusions: impairments such as hypersensitivities or allergies

Exclusion: tolerance to food (b5153)

b 4352   **Functions of lymphatic vessels**
Functions related to vascular channels that transport lymph.

b 4353   **Functions of lymph nodes**
Functions related to glands along the course of lymphatic
vessels.

b 4358   **Immunological system functions, other specified**

b 4359   **Immunological system functions, unspecified**

b 439   **Functions of the haematological and immunological systems, other
specified and unspecified**

Functions of the respiratory system (b440-b449)

b 440   **Respiration functions**
Functions of inhaling air into the lungs, the exchange of gases between
air and blood, and exhaling air.

*Inclusions: functions of respiration rate, rhythm and depth; impairments
such as apnoea, hyperventilation, irregular respiration, paradoxical
respiration, and brochial spasm, and as in pulmonary emphysema*

*Exclusions: respiratory muscle functions (b445); additional respiratory
functions (b450); exercise tolerance functions (b455)*

b 4400   **Respiration rate**
Functions related to the number of breaths taken per minute.

*Inclusions: impairments such as rates that are too fast
(tachypnoea) or too slow (bradypnoea)*

b 4401   **Respiratory rhythm**
Functions related to the periodicity and regularity of breathing.

Inclusions: impairments such as irregular breathing

b 4402   **Depth of respiration**
Functions related to the volume of expansion of the lungs during breathing.

Inclusions: impairments such as superficial or shallow respiration

b 4408   **Respiration functions, other specified**

b 4409   **Respiration functions, unspecified**

b 445   **Respiratory muscle functions**
Functions of the muscles involved in breathing.

Inclusions: functions of thoracic respiratory muscles; functions of the diaphragm; functions of accessory respiratory muscles

Exclusions: respiration functions (b440); additional respiratory functions (b450); exercise tolerance functions (b455)

b 4450   **Functions of the thoracic respiratory muscles**
Functions of the thoracic muscles involved in breathing.

b 4451   **Functions of the diaphragm**
Functions of the diaphragm as involved in breathing.

b 4452   **Functions of accessory respiratory muscles**
Functions of the additional muscles involved in breathing.

b 4458   **Respiratory muscle functions, other specified**

b 4459   **Respiratory muscle functions, unspecified**

b 449   **Functions of the respiratory system, other specified and unspecified**

Additional functions and sensations of the cardiovascular and respiratory systems (b450-b469)

b 450   **Additional respiratory functions**
Additional functions related to breathing, such as coughing, sneezing and yawning.

Inclusions: functions of blowing, whistling and mouth breathing

b455 **Exercise tolerance functions**
Functions related to respiratory and cardiovascular capacity as required for enduring physical exertion.

Inclusions: functions of physical endurance, aerobic capacity, stamina and fatiguability

Exclusions: functions of the cardiovascular system (b410-b429); haematological system functions (b430); respiration functions (b440); respiratory muscle functions (b445); additional respiratory functions (b450)

> **b4550** **General physical endurance**
> Functions related to the general level of tolerance of physical exercise or stamina.
>
> **b4551** **Aerobic capacity**
> Functions related to the extent to which a person can exercise without getting out of breath.
>
> **b4552** **Fatiguability**
> Functions related to susceptibility to fatigue, at any level of exertion.
>
> **b4558** **Exercise tolerance functions, other specified**
>
> **b4559** **Exercise tolerance functions, unspecified**

b460 **Sensations associated with cardiovascular and respiratory functions**
Sensations such as missing a heart beat, palpitation and shortness of breath.

Inclusions: sensations of tightness of chest, feelings of irregular beat, dyspnoea, air hunger, choking, gagging and wheezing

Exclusion: sensation of pain (b280)

b469 **Additional functions and sensations of the cardiovascular and respiratory systems, other specified and unspecified**

b498 **Functions of the cardiovascular, haematological, immunological and respiratory systems, other specified**

b499 **Functions of the cardiovascular, haematological, immunological and respiratory systems, unspecified**

Chapter 5

Functions of the digestive, metabolic and endocrine systems

This chapter is about the functions of ingestion, digestion and elimination, as well as functions involved in metabolism and the endocrine glands.

Functions related to the digestive system (b510-b539)

b510   **Ingestion functions**
Functions related to taking in and manipulating solids or liquids through the mouth into the body.

Inclusions: functions of sucking, chewing and biting, manipulating food in the mouth, salivation, swallowing, burping, regurgitation, spitting and vomiting; impairments such as dysphagia, aspiration of food, aerophagia, excessive salivation, drooling and insufficient salivation

Exclusion: sensations associated with digestive system (b535)

   b5100   **Sucking**
Functions of drawing into the mouth by a suction force produced by movements of the cheeks, lips and tongue.

   b5101   **Biting**
Functions of cutting into, piercing or tearing off food with the front teeth.

   b5102   **Chewing**
Functions of crushing, grinding and masticating food with the back teeth (e.g. molars).

   b5103   **Manipulation of food in the mouth**
Functions of moving food around the mouth with the teeth and tongue.

   b5104   **Salivation**
Function of the production of saliva within the mouth.

b5105   Swallowing
Functions of clearing the food and drink through the oral
cavity, pharynx and oesophagus into the stomach at an
appropriate rate and speed.

*Inclusions: oral, pharyngeal or oesophageal dysphagia;
impairments in oesophageal passage of food*

b51050   Oral swallowing
Function of clearing the food and drink through the
oral cavity at an appropriate rate and speed.

b51051   Pharyngeal swallowing
Function of clearing the food and drink through the
pharynx at an appropriate rate and speed.

b51052   Oesophageal swallowing
Function of clearing the food and drink through the
oesophagus at an appropriate rate and speed.

b51058   Swallowing, other specified

b51059   Swallowing, unspecified

b5106   Regurgitation and vomiting
Functions of moving food or liquid in the reverse direction to
ingestion, from stomach to oesophagus to mouth and out.

b5108   Ingestion functions, other specified

b5109   Ingestion functions, unspecified

b515   **Digestive functions**
Functions of transporting food through the gastrointestinal tract,
breakdown of food and absorption of nutrients.

*Inclusions: functions of transport of food through the stomach, peristalsis;
breakdown of food, enzyme production and action in stomach and
intestines; absorption of nutrients and tolerance to food; impairments
such as in hyperacidity of stomach, malabsorption, intolerance to food,
hypermotility of intestines, intestinal paralysis, intestinal obstruction and
decreased bile production*

*Exclusions: ingestion functions (b510); assimilation functions (b520);
defecation functions (b525); sensations associated with the digestive
system (b535)*

b5150   Transport of food through stomach and intestines
Peristalsis and related functions that mechanically move food
through stomach and intestines.

b5151   Breakdown of food
Functions of mechanically reducing food to smaller particles in
the gastrointestinal tract.

b5152   Absorption of nutrients
Functions of passing food and drink nutrients into the blood
stream from along the intestines.

b5153   Tolerance to food
Functions of accepting suitable food and drink for digestion
and rejecting what is unsuitable.

*Inclusion: impairments such as hypersensitivities, gluten
intolerance*

b5158   Digestive functions, other specified

b5159   Digestive functions, unspecified

b520   Assimilation functions
Functions by which nutrients are converted into components of the
living body.

Inclusion: functions of storage of nutrients in the body

*Exclusions: digestive functions (b515); defecation functions (b525); weight
maintenance functions (b530); general metabolic functions (b540)*

b525   Defecation functions
Functions of elimination of wastes and undigested food as faeces and
related functions.

*Inclusions: functions of elimination, faecal consistency, frequency of
defecation; faecal continence, flatulence; impairments such as
constipation, diarrhoea, watery stool and anal sphincter incompetence or
incontinence*

*Exclusions: digestive functions (b515); assimilation functions (b520);
sensations associated with the digestive system (b535)*

b5250   Elimination of faeces
Functions of the elimination of waste from the rectum,
including the functions of contraction of the abdominal
muscles in doing so.

b 5251   **Faecal consistency**
Consistency of faeces such as hard, firm, soft or watery.

b 5252   **Frequency of defecation**
Functions involved in the frequency of defecation.

b 5253   **Faecal continence**
Functions involved in voluntary control over the elimination
function.

b 5254   **Flatulence**
Functions involved in the expulsion of excessive amounts of air
or gases from the intestines.

b 5258   **Defecation functions, other specified**

b 5259   **Defecation functions, unspecified**

b 530   **Weight maintenance functions**
Functions of maintaining appropriate body weight, including weight
gain during the developmental period.

*Inclusions: functions of maintenance of acceptable Body Mass Index
(BMI); and impairments such as underweight, cachexia, wasting,
overweight, emaciation and such as in primary and secondary obesity*

*Exclusions: assimilation functions (b520); general metabolic functions
(b540); endocrine gland functions (b555)*

b 535   **Sensations associated with the digestive system**
Sensations arising from eating, drinking and related digestive functions.

*Inclusions: sensations of nausea, feeling bloated, and the feeling of
abdominal cramps; fullness of stomach, globus feeling, spasm of stomach,
gas in stomach and heartburn*

*Exclusions: sensation of pain (b280); ingestion functions (b510); digestive
functions (b515); defecation functions (b525)*

b 5350   **Sensation of nausea**
Sensation of needing to vomit.

b 5351   **Feeling bloated**
Sensation of distension of the stomach or abdomen.

    b 5352　**Sensation of abdominal cramp**
         Sensation of spasmodic or painful muscular contractions of the
         smooth muscles of the gastrointestinal tract.

    b 5358　**Sensations associated with the digestive system, other**
         specified

    b 5359　**Sensations associated with the digestive system, unspecified**

b 539　Functions related to the digestive system, other specified and
      unspecified

Functions related to metabolism and the endocrine system (b540-b559)

b 540　General metabolic functions
      Functions of regulation of essential components of the body such as
      carbohydrates, proteins and fats, the conversion of one to another, and
      their breakdown into energy.

      *Inclusions: functions of metabolism, basal metabolic rate, metabolism of
      carbohydrate, protein and fat, catabolism, anabolism, energy production
      in the body; increase or decrease in metabolic rate*

      *Exclusions: assimilation functions (b520); weight maintenance functions
      (b530); water, mineral and electrolyte balance functions (b545);
      thermoregulatory functions (b550); endocrine glands functions (b555)*

    b 5400　**Basal metabolic rate**
         Functions involved in oxygen consumption of the body at
         specified conditions of rest and temperature.

         *Inclusions: increase or decrease in basic metabolic rate;
         impairments such as in hyperthyroidism and hypothyroidism*

    b 5401　**Carbohydrate metabolism**
         Functions involved in the process by which carbohydrates in
         the diet are stored and broken down into glucose and
         subsequently into carbon dioxide and water.

    b 5402　**Protein metabolism**
         Functions involved in the process by which proteins in the diet
         are converted to amino acids and broken down further in the
         body.

b 5403 Fat metabolism
Functions involved in the process by which fat in the diet is
stored and broken down in the body.

b 5408 General metabolic functions, other specified

b 5409 General metabolic functions, unspecified

b 545 Water, mineral and electrolyte balance functions
Functions of the regulation of water, mineral and electrolytes in the
body.

*Inclusions: functions of water balance, balance of minerals such as
calcium, zinc and iron, and balance of electrolytes such as sodium and
potassium; impairments such as in water retention, dehydration,
hypercalcaemia, hypocalcaemia, iron deficiency, hypernatraemia,
hyponatraemia, hyperkalaemia and hypokalaemia*

*Exclusions: haematological system functions (b430); general metabolic
functions (b540); endocrine gland functions (b555)*

b 5450 Water balance
Functions involved in maintaining the level or amount of water
in the body.

Inclusions: impairments such as in dehydration and rehydration

b 54500 Water retention
Functions involved in keeping water in the body.

b 54501 Maintenance of water balance
Functions involved in maintaining the optimal
amount of water in the body.

b 54508 Water balance functions, other specified

b 54509 Water balance functions, unspecified

b 5451 Mineral balance
Functions involved in maintaining an equilibrium between
intake, storage, utilization and excretion of minerals in the
body.

b 5452 Electrolyte balance
Functions involved in maintaining an equilibrium between
intake, storage, utilization and excretion of electrolytes in the
body.

b 5458   Water, mineral and electrolyte balance functions, other specified

b 5459   Water, mineral and electrolyte balance functions, unspecified

b 550   Thermoregulatory functions
Functions of the regulation of body temperature.

Inclusions: functions of maintenance of body temperature; impairments such as hypothermia, hyperthermia

Exclusions: general metabolic functions (b540); endocrine gland functions (b555)

b 5500   Body temperature
Functions involved in regulating the core temperature of the body.

Inclusions: impairments such as hyperthermia or hypothermia

b 5501   Maintenance of body temperature
Functions involved in maintaining optimal body temperature as environmental temperature changes.

Inclusion: tolerance to heat or cold

b 5508   Thermoregulatory functions, other specified

b 5509   Thermoregulatory functions, unspecified

b 555   Endocrine gland functions
Functions of production and regulation of hormonal levels in the body, including cyclical changes.

Inclusions: functions of hormonal balance; hyperpituitarism, hypopituitarism, hyperthyroidism, hypothyroidism, hyperadrenalism, hypoadrenalism, hyperparathyroidism, hypoparathyroidism, hypergonadism, hypogonadism

Exclusions: general metabolic functions (b540); water, mineral and electrolyte balance functions (b545); thermoregulatory functions (b550); sexual functions (b640); menstruation functions (b650)

b 559   Functions related to metabolism and the endocrine system, other specified and unspecified

b 598   Functions of the digestive, metabolic and endocrine systems, other specified

b 599 Functions of the digestive, metabolic and endocrine systems, unspecified

Chapter 6

Genitourinary and reproductive functions

This chapter is about the functions of urination and the reproductive functions, including sexual and procreative functions.

Urinary functions (b610-b639)

b610   **Urinary excretory functions**
Functions of filtration and collection of the urine.

Inclusions: functions of urinary filtration, collection of urine; impairments such as in renal insufficiency, anuria, oliguria, hydronephrosis, hypotonic urinary bladder and ureteric obstruction

Exclusion: urination functions (b620)

> **b6100**   **Filtration of urine**
> Functions of filtration of urine by the kidneys.

> **b6101**   **Collection of urine**
> Functions of collection and storage of urine by the ureters and bladder.

> **b6108**   **Urinary excretory functions, other specified**

> **b6109**   **Urinary excretory functions, unspecified**

b620   **Urination functions**
Functions of discharge of urine from the urinary bladder.

Inclusions: functions of urination, frequency of urination, urinary continence; impairments such as in stress, urge, reflex, overflow, continuous incontinence, dribbling, automatic bladder, polyuria, urinary retention and urinary urgency

Exclusions: urinary excretory functions (b610); sensations associated with urinary functions (b630)

> **b6200**   **Urination**
> Functions of voiding the urinary bladder.
>
> *Inclusions: impairments such as in urine retention*

> **b6201**   **Frequency of urination**
> Functions involved in the number of times urination occurs.

b 6202 **Urinary continence**
Functions of control over urination.

Inclusions:impairments such as in stress, urge, reflex, continuous and mixed incontinence

b 6208 **Urination functions, other specified**

b 6209 **Urination functions, unspecified**

b630 **Sensations associated with urinary functions**
Sensations arising from voiding and related urinary functions

Inclusions: sensations of incomplete voiding of urine, feeling of fullness of bladder

Exclusions: sensations of pain (b280); urination functions (b620)

b639 **Urinary functions, other specified and unspecified**

Genital and reproductive functions (b640-b679)

b640 **Sexual functions**
Mental and physical functions related to the sexual act, including the arousal, preparatory, orgasmic and resolution stages.

Inclusions: functions of the sexual arousal, preparatory, orgasmic and resolution phase: functions related to sexual interest, performance, penile erection, clitoral erection, vaginal lubrication, ejaculation, orgasm; impairments such as impotence, frigidity, vaginismus, premature ejaculation, priapism and delayed ejaculation

Exclusions: procreation functions (b660); sensations associated with genital and reproductive functions (b670)

b 6400 **Functions of sexual arousal phase**
Functions of sexual interest and excitement.

b 6401 **Functions of sexual preparatory phase**
Functions of engaging in sexual intercourse.

b 6402 **Functions of orgasmic phase**
Functions of reaching orgasm.

b 6403   **Functions of sexual resolution phase**
Functions of satisfaction after orgasm and accompanying
relaxation.

Inclusions: impairments such as dissatisfaction with orgasm

b 6408   **Sexual functions, other specified**

b 6409   **Sexual functions, unspecified**

b650   **Menstruation functions**
Functions associated with the menstrual cycle, including regularity of
menstruation and discharge of menstrual fluids.

*Inclusions: functions of regularity and interval of menstruation, extent of
menstrual bleeding, menarche, menopause; impairments such as primary
and secondary amenorrhoea, menorrhagia, polymenorrhoea and
retrograde menstruationpremenstrual tension*

*Exclusions: sexual functions (b640); procreation functions (b660);
sensations associated with genital and reproductive functions (b670);
sensation of pain (b280)*

b 6500   **Regularity of menstrual cycle**
Functions involved in the regularity of the menstrual cycle.

Inclusions: too frequent or too few occurrences of menstruation

b 6501   **Interval between menstruation**
Functions relating to the length of time between two menstrual
cycles.

b 6502   **Extent of menstrual bleeding**
Functions involved in the quantity of menstrual flow.

*Inclusions: too little menstrual flow (hypomenorrhoea); too
much menstrual flow (menorrhagia, hypermenorrhoea)*

b 6508   **Menstruation functions, other specified**

b 6509   **Menstruation functions, unspecified**

b 660   Procreation functions
Functions associated with fertility, pregnancy, childbirth and lactation.

Inclusions: functions of male fertility and female fertility, pregnancy and childbirth, and lactation; impairments such as azoospermia, oligozoospermia, agalactorrhoea, galactorrhoea,alactationand such as in subfertility, sterility, , spontaneous abortions, ectopic pregnancy, miscarriage, small fetus, hydramnios and premature childbirth, and delayed childbirth

Exclusions: sexual functions (b640); menstruation functions (b650)

   b 6600   Functions related to fertility
Functions related to the ability to produce gametes for procreation.

Inclusion: impairments such as in subfertility and sterility

Exclusion: sexual functions (b640)

   b 6601   Functions related to pregnancy
Functions involved in becoming pregnant and being pregnant.

   b 6602   Functions related to childbirth
Functions involved during childbirth.

   b 6603   Lactation
Functions involved in producing milk and making it available to the child.

   b 6608   Procreation functions, other specified

   b 6609   Procreation functions, unspecified

b 670   Sensations associated with genital and reproductive functions
Sensations arising from sexual arousal, intercourse, menstruation, and related genital or reproductive functions.

Inclusions: sensations of dyspareunia, dysmenorrhoea, hot flushes during menopause and night sweats during menopause

Exclusions: sensation of pain (b280); sensations associated with urinary functions (b630); sexual functions (b640); menstruation functions (b650); procreation functions (b660)

   b 6700   Discomfort associated with sexual intercourse
Sensations associated with sexual arousal, preparation, intercourse, orgasm and resolution.

b 6701   Discomfort associated with the menstrual cycle
Sensations involved with menstruation, including pre- and post-menstrual phases.

b 6702   Discomfort associated with menopause
Sensations associated with cessation of the menstrual cycle.

Inclusions: hot flushes and night sweats during menopause

b 6708   Sensations associated with genital and reproductive functions, other specified

b 6709   Sensations associated with genital and reproductive functions, unspecified

b 679   Genital and reproductive functions, other specified and unspecified

b 698   Genitourinary and reproductive functions, other specified

b 699   Genitourinary and reproductive functions, unspecified

Chapter 7
Neuromusculoskeletal and movement-related functions

This chapter is about the functions of movement and mobility, including functions of joints, bones, reflexes and muscles.

Functions of the joints and bones (b710-b729)

b710   **Mobility of joint functions**
Functions of the range and ease of movement of a joint.

Inclusions: functions of mobility of single or several joints, vertebral, shoulder, elbow, wrist, hip, knee, ankle, small joints of hands and feet; mobility of joints generalized; impairments such as in hypermobility of joints, frozen joints, frozen shoulder, arthritis

Exclusions: stability of joint functions (b715); control of voluntary movement functions (b760)

> **b7100**   **Mobility of a single joint**
> Functions of the range and ease of movement of one joint.

> **b7101**   **Mobility of several joints**
> Functions of the range and ease of movement of more than one joint.

> **b7102**   **Mobility of joints generalized**
> Functions of the range and ease of movement of joints throughout the body.

> **b7108**   **Mobility of joint functions, other specified**

> **b7109**   **Mobility of joint functions, unspecified**

b715   **Stability of joint functions**
Functions of the maintenance of structural integrity of the joints.

Inclusions: functions of the stability of a single joint, several joints, and joints generalized; impairments such as in unstable shoulder joint, dislocation of a joint, dislocation of shoulder and hip

Exclusion: mobility of joint functions (b710)

    b 7150   **Stability of a single joint**
Functions of the maintenance of structural integrity of one joint.

    b 7151   **Stability of several joints**
Functions of the maintenance of structural integrity of more than one joint.

    b 7152   **Stability of joints generalized**
Functions of the maintenance of structural integrity of joints throughout the body.

    b 7158   **Stability of joint functions, other specified**

    b 7159   **Stability of joint functions, unspecified**

b 720   **Mobility of bone functions**
Functions of the range and ease of movement of the scapula, pelvis, carpal and tarsal bones.

Inclusions: impairments such as frozen scapula and frozen pelvis

Exclusion: mobility of joints functions (b710)

    b 7200   **Mobility of scapula**
Functions of the range and ease of movement of the scapula.

Inclusions: impairments such as protraction, retraction, laterorotation and medial rotation of the scapula

    b 7201   **Mobility of pelvis**
Functions of the range and ease of movement of the pelvis.

Inclusion: rotation of the pelvis

    b 7202   **Mobility of carpal bones**
Functions of the range and ease of movement of the carpal bones.

    b 7203   **Mobility of tarsal bones**
Functions of the range and ease of movement of the tarsal bones.

    b 7208   **Mobility of bone functions, other specified**

    b 7209   **Mobility of bone functions, specified**

b 729   **Functions of the joints and bones, other specified and unspecified**

Muscle functions (b730-b749)

b730   **Muscle power functions**
Functions related to the force generated by the contraction of a muscle or muscle groups.

Inclusions: functions associated with the power of specific muscles and muscle groups, muscles of one limb, one side of the body, the lower half of the body, all limbs, the trunk and the body as a whole; impairments such as weakness of small muscles in feet and hands, muscle paresis, muscle paralysis, monoplegia, hemiplegia, paraplegia, quadriplegia and akinetic mutism

Exclusions: functions of structures adjoining the eye (b215); muscle tone functions (b735); muscle endurance functions (b740)

     b7300   **Power of isolated muscles and muscle groups**
                   Functions related to the force generated by the contraction of specific and isolated muscles and muscle groups.

                   Inclusions: impairments such as weakness of small muscles of feet or hands

     b7301   **Power of muscles of one limb**
                   Functions related to the force generated by the contraction of the muscles and muscle groups of one arm or leg.

                   Inclusions: impairments such as monoparesis and monoplegia

     b7302   **Power of muscles of one side of the body**
                   Functions related to the force generated by the contraction of the muscles and muscle groups found on the left or right side of the body.

                   Inclusions: impairments such as hemiparesis and hemiplegia

     b7303   **Power of muscles in lower half of the body**
                   Functions related to the force generated by the contraction of the muscles and muscle groups found in the lower half of the body.

                   Inclusions: impairments such as paraparesis and paraplegia

     b7304   **Power of muscles of all limbs**
                   Functions related to the force generated by the contraction of muscles and muscle groups of all four limbs.

                   Inclusions: impairments such as tetraparesis and tetraplegia

b 7305   **Power of muscles of the trunk**
Functions related to the force generated by the contraction of muscles and muscle groups in the trunk.

b 7306   **Power of all muscles of the body**
Functions related to the force generated by the contraction of all muscles and muscle groups of the body.

Inclusions: impairments such as akinetic mutism

b 7308   **Muscle power functions, other specified**

b 7309   **Muscle power functions, unspecified**

b 735   **Muscle tone functions**
Functions related to the tension present in the resting muscles and the resistance offered when trying to move the muscles passively.

Inclusions: functions associated with the tension of isolated muscles and muscle groups, muscles of one limb, one side of the body and the lower half of the body, muscles of all limbs, muscles of the trunk, and all muscles of the body; impairments such as hypotonia, hypertonia and muscle spasticity

Exclusions: muscle power functions (b730); muscle endurance functions (b740)

b 7350   **Tone of isolated muscles and muscle groups**
Functions related to the tension present in the resting isolated muscles and muscle groups and the resistance offered when trying to move those muscles passively.

Inclusions: impairments such as in focal dystonias, e.g. torticollis

b 7351   **Tone of muscles of one limb**
Functions related to the tension present in the resting muscles and muscle groups in one arm or leg and the resistance offered when trying to move those muscles passively.

Inclusions: impairments associated with monoparesis and monoplegia

b 7352   **Tone of muscles of one side of body**
Functions related to the tension present in the resting muscles and muscle groups of the right or left side of the body and the resistance offered when trying to move those muscles passively.

Inclusions: impairments associated with hemiparesis and hemiplegia

b 7353   **Tone of muscles of lower half of body**
Functions related to the tension present in the resting muscles and muscle groups in the lower half of the body and the resistance offered when trying to move those muscles passively.

Inclusions: impairments associated with paraparesis and paraplegia

b 7354   **Tone of muscles of all limbs**
Functions related to the tension present in the resting muscles and muscle groups in all four limbs and the resistance offered when trying to move those muscles passively.

Inclusions: impairments associated with tetraparesis and tetraplegia

b 7355   **Tone of muscles of trunk**
Functions related to the tension present in the resting muscles and muscle groups of the trunk and the resistance offered when trying to move those muscles passively.

b 7356   **Tone of all muscles of the body**
Functions related to the tension present in the resting muscles and muscle groups of the whole body and the resistance offered when trying to move those muscles passively.

Inclusions: impairments such as in generalized dystonias and Parkinson's disease, or general paresis and paralysis

b 7358   **Muscle tone functions, other specified**

b 7359   **Muscle tone functions, unspecified**

b 740   **Muscle endurance functions**
Functions related to sustaining muscle contraction for the required period of time.

Inclusions: functions associated with sustaining muscle contraction for isolated muscles and muscle groups, and all muscles of the body; impairments such as in myasthenia gravis

Exclusions: exercise tolerance functions (b455); muscle power functions (b730); muscle tone functions (b735)

b 7400   **Endurance of isolated muscles**
Functions related to sustaining muscle contraction of isolated muscles for the required period of time.

b 7401   Endurance of muscle groups
Functions related to sustaining muscle contraction of isolated muscle groups for the required period of time.

Inclusions: impairments associated with monoparesis, monoplegia, hemiparesis and hemiplegia, paraparesis and paraplegia

b 7402   Endurance of all muscles of the body
Functions related to sustaining muscle contraction of all muscles of the body for the required period of time.

Inclusions: impairments sddocaited with tetraparesis, tetraplegia, general paresis and paralysis

b 7408   Muscle endurance functions, other specified

b 7409   Muscle endurance functions, unspecified

b 749   **Muscle functions, other specified and unspecified**

Movement functions (b750-b789)

b 750   **Motor reflex functions**
Functions of involuntary contraction of muscles automatically induced by specific stimuli.

Inclusions: functions of stretch motor reflex, automatic local joint reflex, reflexes generated by noxious stimuli and other exteroceptive stimuli; withdrawal reflex, biceps reflex, radius reflex, quadriceps reflex, patellar reflex, ankle reflex

b 7500   Stretch motor reflex
Functions of involuntary contractions of muscles automatically induced by stretching.

b 7501   Reflexes generated by noxious stimuli
Functions of involuntary contractions of muscles automatically induced by painful or other noxious stimuli.

Inclusion: withdrawal reflex

b 7502   Reflexes generated by other exteroceptive stimuli
Functions of involuntary contractions of muscles automatically induced by external stimuli other than noxious stimuli.

b 7508   Motor reflex functions, other specified

b 7509   Motor reflex functions, unspecified

b 755   **Involuntary movement reaction functions**
Functions of involuntary contractions of large muscles or the whole body induced by body position, balance and threatening stimuli.

Inclusions: functions of postural reactions, righting reactions, body adjustment reactions, balance reactions, supporting reactions, defensive reactions

Exclusion: motor reflex functions (b750)

b 760   **Control of voluntary movement functions**
Functions associated with control over and coordination of voluntary movements.

Inclusions: functions of control of simple voluntary movements and of complex voluntary movements, coordination of voluntary movements, supportive functions of arm or leg, right left motor coordination, eye hand coordination, eye foot coordination; impairments such as control and coordination problems, e.g. dysdiadochokinesia

Exclusions: muscle power functions (b730); involuntary movement functions (b765); gait pattern functions (b770)

b 7600   **Control of simple voluntary movements**
Functions associated with control over and coordination of simple or isolated voluntary movements.

b 7601   **Control of complex voluntary movements**
Functions associated with control over and coordination of complex voluntary movements.

b 7602   **Coordination of voluntary movements**
Functions associated with coordination of simple and complex voluntary movements, performing movements in an orderly combination.

Inclusions: right left coordination, coordination of visually directed movements, such as eye hand coordination and eye foot coordination; impairments such as dysdiadochokinesia

b 7603   **Supportive functions of arm or leg**
Functions associated with control over and coordination of voluntary movements by placing weight either on the arms (elbows or hands) or on the legs (knees or feet).

b 7608   **Control of voluntary movement functions, other specified**

b 7609   Control of voluntary movement functions, unspecified

b 765   **Involuntary movement functions**
Functions of unintentional, non- or semi-purposive involuntary
contractions of a muscle or group of muscles.

*Inclusions: involuntary contractions of muscles; impairments such as
tremors, tics, mannerisms, stereotypies, motor perseveration, chorea,
athetosis, vocal tics, dystonic movements and dyskinesia*

*Exclusions: control of voluntary movement functions (b760); gait pattern
functions (b770)*

b 7650   **Involuntary contractions of muscles**
Functions of unintentional, non- or semi-purposive
involuntary contractions of a muscle or group of muscles, such
as those involved as part of a psychological dysfunction.

*Inclusions: impairments such as choreatic and athetotic
movements; sleep-related movement disorders*

b 7651   **Tremor**
Functions of alternating contraction and relaxation of a group
of muscles around a joint, resulting in shakiness.

b 7652   **Tics and mannerisms**
Functions of repetitive, quasi-purposive, involuntary
contractions of a group of muscles.

*Inclusion: impairments such as vocal tics, coprolalia and
bruxism*

b 7653   **Stereotypies and motor perseveration**
Functions of spontaneous, non-purposive movements such as
repetitively rocking back and forth and nodding the head or
wiggling.

b 7658   **Involuntary movement functions, other specified**

b 7659   **Involuntary movement functions, unspecified**

b770 Gait pattern functions

Functions of movement patterns associated with walking, running or other whole body movements.

Inclusions: walking patterns and running patterns; impairments such as spastic gait, hemiplegic gait, paraplegic gait, asymmetric gait, limping and stiff gait pattern

Exclusions: muscle power functions (b730); muscle tone functions (b735); control of voluntary movement functions (b760); involuntary movement functions (b765)

b780 Sensations related to muscles and movement functions

Sensations associated with the muscles or muscle groups of the body and their movement.

Inclusions: sensations of muscle stiffness and tightness of muscles, muscle spasm or constriction, and heaviness of muscles

Exclusion: sensation of pain (b280)

    b7800 Sensation of muscle stiffness
    Sensation of tightness or stiffness of muscles.

    b7801 Sensation of muscle spasm
    Sensation of involuntary contraction of a muscle or a group of muscles.

    b7808 Sensations related to muscles and movement functions, other specified

    b7809 Sensations related to muscles and movement functions, unspecified

b789 Movement functions, other specified and unspecified

b798 Neuromusculoskeletal and movement-related functions, other specified

b799 Neuromusculoskeletal and movement-related functions, unspecified

Chapter 8
Functions of the skin and related structures

This chapter is about the functions of skin, nails and hair.

Functions of the skin (b810-b849)

b810 **Protective functions of the skin**
Functions of the skin for protecting the body from physical, chemical and biological threats.

Inclusions: functions of protecting against the sun and other radiation, photosensitivity, pigmentation, quality of skin; insulating function of skin, callus formation, hardening; impairments such as broken skin, ulcers, bedsores and thinning of skin

Exclusions: repair functions of the skin (b820); other functions of the skin (b830)

b820 **Repair functions of the skin**
Functions of the skin for repairing breaks and other damage to the skin.

Inclusions: functions of scab formation, healing, scarring; bruising and keloid formation

Exclusions: protective functions of the skin (b810); other functions of the skin (b830)

b830 **Other functions of the skin**
Functions of the skin other than protection and repair, such as cooling and sweat secretion.

Inclusions: functions of sweating, glandular functions of the skin and resulting body odour

Exclusions: protective functions of the skin (b810); repair functions of the skin (b820)

b840 **Sensation related to the skin**
Sensations related to the skin such as itching, burning sensation and tingling.

Inclusions: impairments such as pins and needles sensation and crawling sensation

Exclusion: sensation of pain (b280)

b849   Functions of the skin, other specified and unspecified

Functions of the hair and nails (b850-b869)

b850   Functions of hair
Functions of the hair, such as protection, coloration and appearance.

Inclusions: functions of growth of hair, pigmentation of hair, location of hair; impairments such as loss of hair or alopecia

b860   Functions of nails
Functions of the nails, such as protection, scratching and appearance.

Inclusions: growth and pigmentation of nails, quality of nails

b869   Functions of the hair and nails, other specified and unspecified

b898   Functions of the skin and related structures, other specified

b899   Functions of the skin and related structures, unspecified

BODY STRUCTURES

Definitions: **Body structures** *are anatomical parts of the body such as organs, limbs and their components.*

       Impairments *are problems in body function or structure as a significant deviation or loss.*

First qualifier

Generic qualifier with the negative scale used to indicate the extent or magnitude of an impairment:

xxx.0 NO impairment	(none, absent, negligible,…)	0-4 %
xxx.1 MILD impairment	(slight, low,…)	5-24 %
xxx.2 MODERATE impairment	(medium, fair,...)	25-49 %
xxx.3 SEVERE impairment	(high, extreme, …)	50-95 %
xxx.4 COMPLETE impairment	(total,…)	96-100 %
xxx.8 not specified		
xxx.9 not applicable		

Broad ranges of percentages are provided for those cases in which calibrated assessment instruments or other standards are available to quantify the impairment in body structure. For example, when "no impairment" or "complete impairment" in body structure is coded, this scaling may have margin of error of up to 5%. "Moderate impairment" is generally up to half of the scale of total impairment. The percentages are to be calibrated in different domains with reference to population standards as percentiles. For this quantification to be used in a uniform manner, assessment procedures need to be developed through research.

Second qualifier

Used to indicate the nature of the change in the respective body structure:

    0   no change in structure
    1   total absence
    2   partial absence
    3   additional part
    4   aberrant dimensions
    5   discontinuity
    6   deviating position
    7   qualitative changes in structure, including accumulation of fluid
    8   not specified
    9   not applicable

Third qualifier (suggested)

To be developed to indicate localization

0 more than one region
1 right
2 left
3 both sides
4 front
5 back
6 proximal
7 distal
8 not specified
9 not applicable

For a further explanation of coding conventions in ICF, refer to Annex 2.

Chapter 1
Structures of the nervous system

s110 Structure of brain

   s1100   Structure of cortical lobes

        s11000 Frontal lobe

        s11001 Temporal lobe

        s11002 Parietal lobe

        s11003 Occipital lobe

        s11008 Structure of cortical lobes, other specified

        s11009 Structure of cortical lobes, unspecified

   s1101   Structure of midbrain

   s1102   Structure of diencephalon

   s1103   Basal ganglia and related structures

   s1104   Structure of cerebellum

   s1105   Structure of brain stem

        s11050 Medulla oblongata

        s11051 Pons

        s11058 Structure of brain stem, other specified

        s11059 Structure of brain stem, unspecified

   s1106   Structure of cranial nerves

   s1108   Structure of brain, other specified

   s1109   Structure of brain, unspecified

s120 Spinal cord and related structures

   s1200   Structure of spinal cord

        s12000 Cervical spinal cord

        s12001 Thoracic spinal cord

           s 12002   Lumbosacral spinal cord

           s 12003   Cauda equina

           s 12008   Structure of spinal cord, other specified

           s 12009   Structure of spinal cord, unspecified

     s 1201   Spinal nerves

     s 1208   Spinal cord and related structures, other specified

     s 1209   Spinal cord and related structures, unspecified

s 130   Structure of meninges

s 140   Structure of sympathetic nervous system

s 150   Structure of parasympathetic nervous system

s 198   Structure of the nervous system, other specified

s 199   Structure of the nervous system, unspecified

Chapter 2
The eye, ear and related structures

s 210   Structure of eye socket

s 220   Structure of eyeball

     s 2200   Conjunctiva, sclera, choroid

     s 2201   Cornea

     s 2202   Iris

     s 2203   Retina

     s 2204   Lens of eyeball

     s 2205   Vitreous body

     s 2208   Structure of eyeball, other specified

     s 2209   Structure of eyeball, unspecified

s 230   Structures around eye

     s 2300   Lachrymal gland and related structures

     s 2301   Eyelid

     s 2302   Eyebrow

     s 2303   External ocular muscles

     s 2308   Structures around eye, other specified

     s 2309   Structures around eye, unspecified

s 240   Structure of external ear

s 250   Structure of middle ear

     s 2500   Tympanic membrane

     s 2501   Eustachian canal

     s 2502   Ossicles

     s 2508   Structure of middle ear, other specified

s 2509   Structure of middle ear, unspecified

s 260   Structure of inner ear

s 2600   Cochlea

s 2601   Vestibular labyrinth

s 2602   Semicircular canals

s 2603   Internal auditory meatus

s 2608   Structure of inner ear, other specified

s 2609   Structure of inner ear, unspecified

s 298   Eye, ear and related structures, other specified

s 299   Eye, ear and related structures, unspecified

Chapter 3
Structures involved in voice and speech

s310   Structure of nose

    s3100   External nose

    s3101   Nasal septum

    s3102   Nasal fossae

    s3108   Structure of nose, other specified

    s3109   Structure of nose, unspecified

s320   Structure of mouth

    s3200   Teeth

    s3201   Gums

    s3202   Structure of palate

        s32020   Hard palate

        s32021   Soft palate

    s3203   Tongue

    s3204   Structure of lips

        s32040   Upper lip

        s32041   Lower lip

    s3208   Structure of mouth, other specified

    s3209   Structure of mouth, unspecified

s330   Structure of pharynx

    s3300   Nasal pharynx

    s3301   Oral pharynx

    s3308   Structure of pharynx, other specified

    s3309   Structure of pharynx, unspecified

s 340 Structure of larynx

    s 3400   Vocal folds

    s 3408   Structure of larynx, other specified

    s 3409   Structure of larynx, unspecified

s 398 Structures involved in voice and speech, other specified

s 399 Structures involved in voice and speech, unspecified

Chapter 4
Structures of the cardiovascular, immunological and respiratory systems

s410 Structure of cardiovascular system

    s4100 Heart

        s41000 Atria

        s41001 Ventricles

        s41008 Structure of heart, other specified

        s41009 Structure of heart, unspecified

    s4101 Arteries

    s4102 Veins

    s4103 Capillaries

    s4108 Structure of cardiovascular system, other specified

    s4109 Structure of cardiovascular system, unspecified

s420 Structure of immune system

    s4200 Lymphatic vessels

    s4201 Lymphatic nodes

    s4202 Thymus

    s4203 Spleen

    s4204 Bone marrow

    s4208 Structure of immune system, other specified

    s4209 Structure of immune system, unspecified

s430 Structure of respiratory system

    s4300 Trachea

s 4301   Lungs

s 43010   Bronchial tree

s 43011   Alveoli

s 43018   Structure of lungs, other specified

s 43019   Structure of lungs, unspecified

s 4302   Thoracic cage

s 4303   Muscles of respiration

s 43030   Intercostal muscles

s 43031   Diaphragm

s 43038   Muscles of respiration, other specified

s 43039   Muscles of respiration, unspecified

s 4308   Structure of respiratory system, other specified

s 4309   Structure of respiratory system, unspecified

s 498   Structures of the cardiovascular, immunological and respiratory systems, other specified

s 499   Structures of the cardiovascular, immunological and respiratory systems, unspecified

Chapter 5
Structures related to the digestive, metabolic and endocrine systems

s510   Structure of salivary glands

s520   Structure of oesophagus

s530   Structure of stomach

s540   Structure of intestine

  s 5400   Small intestine

  s 5401   Large intestine

  s 5408   Structure of intestine, other specified

  s 5409   Structure of intestine, unspecified

s550   Structure of pancreas

s560   Structure of liver

s570   Structure of gall bladder and ducts

s580   Structure of endocrine glands

  s 5800   Pituitary gland

  s 5801   Thyroid gland

  s 5802   Parathyroid gland

  s 5803   Adrenal gland

  s 5808   Structure of endocrine glands, other specified

  s 5809   Structure of endocrine glands, unspecified

s598   Structures related to the digestive, metabolic and endocrine systems, other specified

s599   Structures related to the digestive, metabolic and endocrine systems, unspecified

Chapter 6
Structures related to the genitourinary and reproductive systems

s610 Structure of urinary system

    s6100 Kidneys

    s6101 Ureters

    s6102 Urinary bladder

    s6103 Urethra

    s6108 Structure of urinary system, other specified

    s6109 Structure of urinary system, unspecified

s620 Structure of pelvic floor

s630 Structure of reproductive system

    s6300 Ovaries

    s6301 Structure of uterus

        s63010 Body of uterus

        s63011 Cervix

        s63012 Fallopian tubes

        s63018 Structure of uterus, other specified

        s63019 Structure of uterus, unspecified

    s6302 Breast and nipple

    s6303 Structure of vagina and external genitalia

        s63030 Clitoris

        s63031 Labia majora

        s63032 Labia minora

        s63033 Vaginal canal

    s 6304   Testes

    s 6305   Structure of the penis

        s 63050 Glans penis

        s 63051 Shaft of penis

        s 63058 Structure of penis, other specified

        s 63059 Structure of penis, unspecified

    s 6306   Prostate

    s 6308   Structures of reproductive system, other specified

    s 6309   Structures of reproductive system, unspecified

s 698   Structures related to the genitourinary and reproductive systems, other specified

s 699   Structures related to the genitourinary and reproductive systems, unspecified

Chapter 7
Structures related to movement

s 710   Structure of head and neck region

     s 7100   Bones of cranium

     s 7101   Bones of face

     s 7102   Bones of neck region

     s 7103   Joints of head and neck region

     s 7104   Muscles of head and neck region

     s 7105   Ligaments and fasciae of head and neck region

     s 7108   Structure of head and neck region, other specified

     s 7109   Structure of head and neck region, unspecified

s 720   Structure of shoulder region

     s 7200   Bones of shoulder region

     s 7201   Joints of shoulder region

     s 7202   Muscles of shoulder region

     s 7203   Ligaments and fasciae of shoulder region

     s 7208   Structure of shoulder region, other specified

     s 7209   Structure of shoulder region, unspecified

s 730   Structure of upper extremity

     s 7300   Structure of upper arm

         s 73000   Bones of upper arm

         s 73001   Elbow joint

         s 73002   Muscles of upper arm

         s 73003   Ligaments and fasciae of upper arm

         s 73008   Structure of upper arm, other specified

s 73009   Structure of upper arm, unspecified

s 7301   Structure of forearm

s 73010   Bones of forearm

s 73011   Wrist joint

s 73012   Muscles of forearm

s 73013   Ligaments and fasciae of forearm

s 73018   Structure of forearm, other specified

s 73019   Structure of forearm, unspecified

s 7302   Structure of hand

s 73020   Bones of hand

s 73021   Joints of hand and fingers

s 73022   Muscles of hand

s 73023   Ligaments and fasciae of hand

s 73028   Structure of hand, other specified

s 73029   Structure of hand, unspecified

s 7308   Structure of upper extremity, other specified

s 7309   Structure of upper extremity, unspecified

s 740   Structure of pelvic region

s 7400   Bones of pelvic region

s 7401   Joints of pelvic region

s 7402   Muscles of pelvic region

s 7403   Ligaments and fasciae of pelvic region

s 7408   Structure of pelvic region, other specified

s 7409   Structure of pelvic region, unspecified

s 750   Structure of lower extremity

s 7500   Structure of thigh

s 75000 Bones of thigh

s 75001 Hip joint

s 75002 Muscles of thigh

s 75003 Ligaments and fasciae of thigh

s 75008 Structure of thigh, other specified

s 75009 Structure of thigh, unspecified

s 7501 Structure of lower leg

s 75010 Bones of lower leg

s 75011 Knee joint

s 75012 Muscles of lower leg

s 75013 Ligaments and fasciae of lower leg

s 75018 Structure of lower leg, other specified

s 75019 Structure of lower leg, unspecified

s 7502 Structure of ankle and foot

s 75020 Bones of ankle and foot

s 75021 Ankle joint and joints of foot and toes

s 75022 Muscles of ankle and foot

s 75023 Ligaments and fasciae of ankle and foot

s 75028 Structure of ankle and foot, other specified

s 75029 Structure of ankle and foot, unspecified

s 7508 Structure of lower extremity, other specified

s 7509 Structure of lower extremity, unspecified

s 760 Structure of trunk

s 7600 Structure of vertebral column

s 76000 Cervical vertebral column

s 76001 Thoracic vertebral column

s 76002   Lumbar vertebral column

s 76003   Sacral vertebral column

s 76004   Coccyx

s 76008   Structure of vertebral column, other specified

s 76009   Structure of vertebral column, specified

s 7601   Muscles of trunk

s 7602   Ligaments and fasciae of trunk

s 7608   Structure of trunk, other specified

s 7609   Structure of trunk, unspecified

s 770   Additional musculoskeletal structures related to movement

s 7700   Bones

s 7701   Joints

s 7702   Muscles

s 7703   Extra-articular ligaments, fasciae, extramuscular aponeuroses, retinacula, septa, bursae, unspecified

s 7708   Additional musculoskeletal structures related to movement, other specified

s 7709   Additional musculoskeletal structures related to movement, unspecified

s 798   Structures related to movement, other specified

s 799   Structures related to movement, unspecified

Chapter 8
Skin and related structures

s 810   Structure of areas of skin

    s 8100   Skin of head and neck region

    s 8101   Skin of the shoulder region

    s 8102   Skin of upper extremity

    s 8103   Skin of pelvic region

    s 8104   Skin of lower extremity

    s 8105   Skin of trunk and back

    s 8108   Structure of areas of skin, other specified

    s 8109   Structure of areas of skin, unspecified

s 820   Structure of skin glands

    s 8200   Sweat glands

    s 8201   Sebaceous glands

    s 8208   Structure of skin glands, other specified

    s 8209   Structure of skin glands, unspecified

s 830   Structure of nails

    s 8300   Finger nails

    s 8301   Toe nails

    s 8308   Structure of nails, other specified

    s 8309   Structure of nails, unspecified

s 840   Structure of hair

s 898   Skin and related structures, other specified

s 899   Skin and related structures, unspecifed

ACTIVITIES AND PARTICIPATION

Definitions: *Activity* is the execution of a task or action by an individual.

Participation is involvement in a life situation.

Activity limitations are difficulties an individual may have in executing activities.

Participation restrictions are problems an individual may experience in involvement in life situations.

Qualifiers

The domains for the Activities and Participation component are given in a single list that covers the full range of life areas (from basic learning and watching to composite areas such as social tasks). This component can be used to denote activities (a) or participation (p) or both.

The two qualifiers for the Activities and Participation component are the *performance* qualifier and the *capacity* qualifier. The performance qualifier describes what an individual does in his or her current environment. Because the current environment brings in a societal context, performance as recorded by this qualifier can also be understood as "involvement in a life situation" or "the lived experience" of people in the actual context in which they live. This context includes the environmental factors – all aspects of the physical, social and attitudinal world, which can be coded using the Environmental Factors component.

The capacity qualifier describes an individual's ability to execute a task or an action. This qualifier identifies the highest probable level of functioning that a person may reach in a given domain at a given moment. Capacity is measured in a uniform or standard environment, and thus reflects the environmentally adjusted ability of the individual. The Environmental Factors component can be used to describe the features of this uniform or standard environment.

Both capacity and performance qualifiers can be used both with and without assistive devices or personal assistance, and in accordance with the following scale:

xxx.0 NO difficulty	(none, absent, negligible,…)	0-4 %
xxx.1 MILD difficulty	(slight, low,…)	5-24 %
xxx.2 MODERATE difficulty	(medium, fair,…)	25-49 %
xxx.3 SEVERE difficulty	(high, extreme, …)	50-95 %
xxx.4 COMPLETE difficulty	(total,…)	96-100 %
xxx.8 not specified		
xxx.9 not applicable		

Broad ranges of percentages are provided for those cases in which calibrated assessment instruments or other standards are available to quantify the performance problem or capacity limitation. For example, when no performance problem or a complete performance problem is coded, this scaling has a margin of error of up to 5%. A moderate performance problem is defined as up to half of the scale of a total performance problem. The percentages are to be calibrated in different domains with reference to population standards as percentiles. For this quantification to be used in a uniform manner, assessment procedures need to be developed through research.

For a further explanation of coding convention in ICF, refer to Annex 2.

Chapter 1
Learning and applying knowledge

This chapter is about learning, applying the knowledge that is learned, thinking, solving problems, and making decisions.

Purposeful sensory experiences (d110-d129)

d110 **Watching**
Using the sense of seeing intentionally to experience visual stimuli, such as watching a sporting event or children playing.

d115 **Listening**
Using the sense of hearing intentionally to experience auditory stimuli, such as listening to a radio, music or a lecture.

d120 **Other purposeful sensing**
Using the body's other basic senses intentionally to experience stimuli, such as touching and feeling textures, tasting sweets or smelling flowers.

d129 **Purposeful sensory experiences, other specified and unspecified**

Basic learning (d130-d159)

d130 **Copying**
Imitating or mimicking as a basic component of learning, such as copying a gesture, a sound or the letters of an alphabet.

d135 **Rehearsing**
Repeating a sequence of events or symbols as a basic component of learning, such as counting by tens or practising the recitation of a poem.

d140 **Learning to read**
Developing the competence to read written material (including Braille) with fluency and accuracy, such as recognizing characters and alphabets, sounding out words with correct pronunciation, and understanding words and phrases.

d145 **Learning to write**
Developing the competence to produce symbols that represent sounds, words or phrases in order to convey meaning (including Braille writing), such as spelling effectively and using correct grammar.

d150 Learning to calculate
Developing the competence to manipulate numbers and perform simple and complex mathematical operations, such as using mathematical signs for addition and subtraction and applying the correct mathematical operation to a problem.

d155 Acquiring skills
Developing basic and complex competencies in integrated sets of actions or tasks so as to initiate and follow through with the acquisition of a skill, such as manipulating tools or playing games like chess.

Inclusions: acquiring basic and complex skills

  d1550 Acquiring basic skills
  Learning elementary, purposeful actions, such as learning to manipulate eating utensils, a pencil or a simple tool.

  d1551 Acquiring complex skills
  Learning integrated sets of actions so as to follow rules, and to sequence and coordinate one's movements, such as learning to play games like football or to use a building tool.

  d1558 Acquiring skills, other specified

  d1559 Acquiring skills, unspecified

d159 Basic learning, other specified and unspecified

Applying knowledge (d160-d179)

d160 Focusing attention
Intentionally focusing on specific stimuli, such as by filtering out distracting noises.

d163 Thinking
Formulating and manipulating ideas, concepts, and images, whether goal-oriented or not, either alone or with others, such as creating fiction, proving a theorem, playing with ideas, brainstorming, meditating, pondering, speculating, or reflecting.

Exclusions: solving problems (d175); making decisions (d177)

d166 **Reading**
Performing activities involved in the comprehension and interpretation of written language (e.g. books, instructions or newspapers in text or Braille), for the purpose of obtaining general knowledge or specific information.

Exclusion: learning to read (d140)

d170 **Writing**
Using or producing symbols or language to convey information, such as producing a written record of events or ideas or drafting a letter.

Exclusion: learning to write (d145)

d172 **Calculating**
Performing computations by applying mathematical principles to solve problems that are described in words and producing or displaying the results, such as computing the sum of three numbers or finding the result of dividing one number by another.

Exclusion: learning to calculate (d150)

d175 **Solving problems**
Finding solutions to questions or situations by identifying and analysing issues, developing options and solutions, evaluating potential effects of solutions, and executing a chosen solution, such as in resolving a dispute between two people.

Inclusions: solving simple and complex problems

Exclusions: thinking (d163); making decisions (d177)

d1750 **Solving simple problems**
Finding solutions to a simple problem involving a single issue or question, by identifying and analysing the issue, developing solutions, evaluating the potential effects of the solutions and executing a chosen solution.

d1751 **Solving complex problems**
Finding solutions to a complex problem involving multiple and interrelated issues, or several related problems, by identifying and analysing the issue, developing solutions, evaluating the potential effects of the solutions and executing a chosen solution.

d1758 **Solving problems, other specified**

d1759 **Solving problems, unspecified**

d177 Making decisions
Making a choice among options, implementing the choice, and evaluating the effects of the choice, such as selecting and purchasing a specific item, or deciding to undertake and undertaking one task from among several tasks that need to be done.

Exclusions: thinking (d163); solving problems (d175)

d179 Applying knowledge, other specified and unspecified

d198 Learning and applying knowledge, other specified

d199 Learning and applying knowledge, unspecified

Chapter 2
General tasks and demands

This chapter is about general aspects of carrying out single or multiple tasks, organizing routines and handling stress. These items can be used in conjunction with more specific tasks or actions to identify the underlying features of the execution of tasks under different circumstances.

d210 **Undertaking a single task**
Carrying out simple or complex and coordinated actions related to the mental and physical components of a single task, such as initiating a task, organizing time, space and materials for a task, pacing task performance, and carrying out, completing, and sustaining a task.

Inclusions: undertaking a simple or complex task; undertaking a single task independently or in a group

Exclusions: acquiring skills (d155); solving problems (d175); making decisions (d177); undertaking multiple tasks (d220)

d2100   **Undertaking a simple task**
Preparing, initiating and arranging the time and space required for a simple task; executing a simple task with a single major component, such as reading a book, writing a letter, or making one's bed.

d2101   **Undertaking a complex task**
Preparing, initiating and arranging the time and space for a single complex task; executing a complex task with more than one component, which may be carried out in sequence or simultaneously, such as arranging the furniture in one's home or completing an assignment for school.

d2102   **Undertaking a single task independently**
Preparing, initiating and arranging the time and space for a simple or complex task; managing and executing a task on one's own and without the assistance of others.

d2103   **Undertaking a single task in a group**
Preparing, initiating and arranging the time and space for a single task, simple or complex; managing and executing a task with people who are involved in some or all steps of the task.

d2108   **Undertaking single tasks, other specified**

d2109   **Undertaking single tasks, unspecified**

d 220   Undertaking multiple tasks
Carrying out simple or complex and coordinated actions as components of multiple, integrated and complex tasks in sequence or simultaneously.

Inclusions: undertaking multiple tasks; completing multiple tasks; undertaking multiple tasks independently and in a group

Exclusions: acquiring skills (d155); solving problems (d175); making decisions (d177); undertaking a single task (d210)

d 2200   Carrying out multiple tasks
Preparing, initiating and arranging the time and space needed for several tasks, and managing and executing several tasks, together or sequentially.

d 2201   Completing multiple tasks
Completing several tasks, together or sequentially.

d 2202   Undertaking multiple tasks independently
Preparing, initiating and arranging the time and space for multiple tasks, and managing and executing several tasks together or sequentially, on one's own and without the assistance of others.

d 2203   Undertaking multiple tasks in a group
Preparing, initiating and arranging the time and space for multiple tasks, and managing and executing several tasks together or sequentially with others who are involved in some or all steps of the multiple tasks.

d 2208   Undertaking multiple tasks, other specified

d 2209   Undertaking multiple tasks, unspecified

d 230   Carrying out daily routine
Carrying out simple or complex and coordinated actions in order to plan, manage and complete the requirements of day-to-day procedures or duties, such as budgeting time and making plans for separate activities throughout the day.

Inclusions: managing and completing the daily routine; managing one's own activity level

Exclusion: undertaking multiple tasks (d220)

d2301   Managing daily routine
Carrying out simple or complex and coordinated actions in order to plan and manage the requirements of day-to-day procedures or duties.

d2302   Completing the daily routine
Carrying out simple or complex and coordinated actions in order to complete the requirements of day-to-day procedures or duties.

d2303   Managing one's own activity level
Carrying out actions and behaviours to arrange the requirements in energy and time day-to-day procedures or duties.

d2308   Carrying out daily routine, other specified

d2309   Carrying out daily routine, unspecified

d240   Handling stress and other psychological demands
Carrying out simple or complex and coordinated actions to manage and control the psychological demands required to carry out tasks demanding significant responsibilities and involving stress, distraction, or crises, such as driving a vehicle during heavy traffic or taking care of many children.

Inclusions: handling responsibilities; handling stress and crisis

d2400   Handling responsibilities
Carrying out simple or complex and coordinated actions to manage the duties of task performance and to assess the requirements of these duties.

d2401   Handling stress
Carrying out simple or complex and coordinated actions to cope with pressure, emergencies or stress associated with task performance.

d2402   Handling crisis
Carrying out simple or complex and coordinated actions to cope with decisive turning points in a situation or times of acute danger or difficulty.

d2408   Handling stress and other psychological demands, other specified

      d 2409   Handling stress and other psychological demands, unspecified

d 298   General tasks and demands, other specified

d 299   General tasks and demands, unspecified

Chapter 3
Communication

This chapter is about general and specific features of communicating by language, signs and symbols, including receiving and producing messages, carrying on conversations, and using communication devices and techniques.

Communicating - receiving (d310-d329)

d310 **Communicating with - receiving - spoken messages**
Comprehending literal and implied meanings of messages in spoken language, such as understanding that a statement asserts a fact or is an idiomatic expression.

d315 **Communicating with - receiving - nonverbal messages**
Comprehending the literal and implied meanings of messages conveyed by gestures, symbols and drawings, such as realizing that a child is tired when she rubs her eyes or that a warning bell means that there is a fire.

Inclusions: communicating with - receiving - body gestures, general signs and symbols, drawings and photographs

d3150   **Communicating with - receiving - body gestures**
Comprehending the meaning conveyed by facial expressions, hand movements or signs, body postures, and other forms of body language.

d3151   **Communicating with - receiving - general signs and symbols**
Comprehending the meaning represented by public signs and symbols, such as traffic signs, warning symbols, musical or scientific notations, and icons.

d3152   **Communicating with - receiving - drawings and photographs**
Comprehending the meaning represented by drawings (e.g. line drawings, graphic designs, paintings, three-dimensional representations), graphs, charts and photographs, such as understanding that an upward line on a height chart indicates that a child is growing.

d3158   **Communicating with - receiving - nonverbal messages, other specified**

d3159   **Communicating with - receiving - nonverbal messages, unspecified**

d320   **Communicating with - receiving - formal sign language messages**
Receiving and comprehending messages in formal sign language with literal and implied meaning.

d325   **Communicating with - receiving - written messages**
Comprehending the literal and implied meanings of messages that are conveyed through written language (including Braille), such as following political events in the daily newspaper or understanding the intent of religious scripture.

d329   **Communicating - receiving, other specified and unspecified**

Communicating - producing (d330-d349)

d330   Speaking
Producing words, phrases and longer passages in spoken messages with literal and implied meaning, such as expressing a fact or telling a story in oral language.

d335   **Producing nonverbal messages**
Using gestures, symbols and drawings to convey messages, such as shaking one's head to indicate disagreement or drawing a picture or diagram to convey a fact or complex idea.

Inclusions: producing body gestures, signs, symbols, drawings and photographs

d3350   **Producing body language**
Conveying meaning by movements of the body, such as facial gestures (e.g. smiling, frowning, wincing), arm and hand movements, and postures (e.g. such as embracing to indicate affection).

d3351   **Producing signs and symbols**
Conveying meaning by using signs and symbols (e.g. icons, Bliss board, scientific symbols) and symbolic notation systems, such as using musical notation to convey a melody.

d3352   **Producing drawings and photographs**
Conveying meaning by drawing, painting, sketching, and making diagrams, pictures or photographs, such as drawing a map to give someone directions to a location.

d3358   **Producing nonverbal messages, other specified**

d3359   **Producing nonverbal messages, unspecified**

d340   **Producing messages in formal sign language**
Conveying, with formal sign language, literal and implied meaning.

d345   **Writing messages**
Producing the literal and implied meanings of messages that are
conveyed through written language, such as writing a letter to a friend.

d349   Communication - producing, other specified and unspecified

Conversation and use of communication devices and techniques (d350-d369)

d350   Conversation
Starting, sustaining and ending an interchange of thoughts and ideas,
carried out by means of spoken, written, sign or other forms of
language, with one or more people one knows or who are strangers, in
formal or casual settings.

*Inclusions: starting, sustaining and ending a conversation; conversing
with one or many people*

d3500   **Starting a conversation**
Beginning a dialogue or interchange, such as by introducing
oneself, expressing customary greetings, and introducing a
topic or asking questions.

d3501   **Sustaining a conversation**
Continuing and shaping a dialogue or interchange by adding
ideas, introducing a new topic or retrieving a topic that has
been previously mentioned, as well as by taking turns in
speaking or signing.

d3502   **Ending a conversation**
Finishing a dialogue or interchange with customary
termination statements or expressions and by bringing closure
to the topic under discussion.

d3503   **Conversing with one person**
Initiating, maintaining, shaping and terminating a dialogue or
interchange with one person, such as in discussing the weather
with a friend.

d 3504   Conversing with many people
Initiating, maintaining, shaping and terminating a dialogue or
interchange with more than one individual, such as in starting
and participating in a group interchange.

d 3508   Conversation, other specified

d 3509   Conversation, unspecified

d 355   Discussion
Starting, sustaining and ending an examination of a matter, with
arguments for or against, or debate carried out by means of spoken,
written, sign or other forms of language, with one or more people one
knows or who are strangers, in formal or casual settings.

Inclusion: discussion with one person or many people

d 3550   Discussion with one person
Initiating, maintaining, shaping or terminating an argument or
debate with one person.

d 3551   Discussion with many people
Initiating, maintaining, shaping or terminating an argument or
debate with more than one individual.

d 3558   Discussion, other specified

d 3559   Discussion, unspecified

d 360   Using communication devices and techniques
Using devices, techniques and other means for the purposes of
communicating, such as calling a friend on the telephone.

*Inclusions: using telecommunication devices, using writing machines and
communication techniques*

d 3600   Using telecommunication devices
Using telephones and other machines, such as facsimile or telex
machines, as a means of communication.

d 3601   Using writing machines
Using machines for writing, such as typewriters, computers
and Braille writers, as a means of communication.

d 3602   Using communication techniques
Performing actions and tasks involved in techniques for
communicating, such as reading lips.

d 3608   Using communication devices and techniques, other
          specified

d 3609   Using communication devices and techniques, unspecified

d 369 Conversation and use of communication devices and techniques,
          other specified and unspecified

d 398 Communication, other specified

d 399 Communication, unspecified

Chapter 4
Mobility

This chapter is about moving by changing body position or location or by transferring from one place to another, by carrying, moving or manipulating objects, by walking, running or climbing, and by using various forms of transportation.

Changing and maintaining body position (d410-d429)

d410 **Changing basic body position**

Getting into and out of a body position and moving from one location to another, such as getting up out of a chair to lie down on a bed, and getting into and out of positions of kneeling or squatting.

Inclusion: changing body position from lying down, from squatting or kneeling, from sitting or standing, bending and shifting the body's centre of gravity

Exclusion: transferring oneself (d420)

d4100 **Lying down**

Getting into and out of a lying down position or changing body position from horizonal to any other position, such as standing up or sitting down.

Inclusion: getting into a prostrate position

d4101 **Squatting**

Getting into and out of the seated or crouched posture on one's haunches with knees closely drawn up or sitting on one's heels, such as may be necessary in toilets that are at floor level, or changing body position from squatting to any other position, such as standing up.

d4102 **Kneeling**

Getting into and out of a position where the body is supported by the knees with legs bent, such as during prayers, or changing body position from kneeling to any other position, such as standing up.

d 4103   Sitting

Getting into and out of a seated position and changing body position from sitting down to any other position, such as standing up or lying down.

Inclusions: getting into a sitting position with bent legs or cross-legged; getting into a sitting position with feet supported or unsupported

d 4104   Standing

Getting into and out of a standing position or changing body position from standing to any other position, such as lying down or sitting down.

d 4105   Bending

Tilting the back downwards or to the side, at the torso, such as in bowing or reaching down for an object.

d 4106   Shifting the body's centre of gravity

Adjusting or moving the weight of the body from one position to another while sitting, standing or lying, such as moving from one foot to another while standing.

Exclusions: transferring oneself (d420); walking (d450)

d 4108   Changing basic body position, other specified

d 4109   Changing basic body position, unspecified

d 415   Maintaining a body position

Staying in the same body position as required, such as remaining seated or remaining standing for work or school.

Inclusions: maintaining a lying, squatting, kneeling, sitting and standing position

d 4150   Maintaining a lying position

Staying in a lying position for some time as required, such as remaining in a prone position in a bed.

Inclusions: staying in a prone (face down or prostrate), supine (face upwards) or side-lying position

d 4151   Maintaining a squatting position

Staying in a squatting position for some time as required, such as when sitting on the floor without a seat.

d 4152   Maintaining a kneeling position

Staying in a kneeling position where the body is supported by the knees with legs bent for some time as required, such as during prayers in church.

d 4153   Maintaining a sitting position

Staying in a seated position, on a seat or the floor, for some time as required, such as when sitting at a desk or table.

Inclusions: staying in a sitting position with straight legs or cross-legged, with feet supported or unsupported

d 4154   Maintaining a standing position

Staying in a standing position for some time as required, such as when standing in a queue.

Inclusions: staying in a standing position on a slope, on slippery or hard surfaces

d 4158   Maintaining a body position, other specified

d 4159   Maintaining a body position, unspecified

d 420   Transferring oneself

Moving from one surface to another, such as sliding along a bench or moving from a bed to a chair, without changing body position.

Inclusions: transferring oneself while sitting or lying

Exclusion: changing basic body position (d410)

d 4200   Transferring oneself while sitting

Moving from a sitting position on one seat to another seat on the same or a different level, such as moving from a chair to a bed.

Inclusions: moving from a chair to another seat, such as a toilet seat; moving from a wheelchair to a car seat

Exclusion: changing basic body position (d410)

d 4201   Transferring oneself while lying

Moving from one lying position to another on the same or a different level, such as moving from one bed to another.

Exclusion: changing basic body position (d410)

d 4208   Transferring oneself, other specified

d 4209   Transferring oneself, unspecified

d429   Changing and maintaining body position, other specified and unspecified

Carrying, moving and handling objects (d430-d449)

d430   Lifting and carrying objects
Raising up an object or taking something from one place to another, such as when lifting a cup or carrying a child from one room to another.

Inclusions: lifting, carrying in the hands or arms, or on shoulders, hip, back or head; putting down

   d4300   **Lifting**
Raising up an object in order to move it from a lower to a higher level, such as when lifting a glass from the table.

   d4301   **Carrying in the hands**
Taking or transporting an object from one place to another using the hands, such as when carrying a drinking glass or a suitcase.

   d4302   **Carrying in the arms**
Taking or transporting an object from one place to another using the arms and hands, such as when carrying a child.

   d4303   **Carrying on shoulders, hip and back**
Taking or transporting an object from one place to another using the shoulders, hip or back, or some combination of these, such as when carrying a large parcel.

   d4304   **Carrying on the head**
Taking or transporting an object from one place to another using the head, such when as carrying a container of water on the head.

   d4305   **Putting down objects**
Using hands, arms or other parts of the body to place an object down on a surface or place, such as when lowering a container of water to the ground.

   d4308   **Lifting and carrying, other specified**

   d4309   **Lifting and carrying, unspecified**

d435   **Moving objects with lower extremities**

Performing coordinated actions aimed at moving an object by using the legs and feet, such as kicking a ball or pushing pedals on a bicycle.

Inclusions: pushing with lower extremities; kicking

    d4350   **Pushing with lower extremities**

Using the legs and feet to exert a force on an object to move it away, such as pushing a chair away with a foot.

    d4351   **Kicking**

Using the legs and feet to propel something away, such as kicking a ball.

    d4358   **Moving objects with lower extremities, other specified**

    d4359   **Moving objects with lower extremities, unspecified**

d440   **Fine hand use**

Performing the coordinated actions of handling objects, picking up, manipulating and releasing them using one's hand, fingers and thumb, such as required to lift coins off a table or turn a dial or knob.

Inclusions: picking up, grasping, manipulating and releasing

Exclusion: lifting and carrying objects (d430)

    d4400   **Picking up**

Lifting or taking up a small object with hands and fingers, such as when picking up a pencil.

    d4401   **Grasping**

Using one or both hands to seize and hold something, such as when grasping a tool or a door knob.

    d4402   **Manipulating**

Using fingers and hands to exert control over, direct or guide something, such as when handling coins or other small objects.

    d4403   **Releasing**

Using fingers and hands to let go or set free something so that it falls or changes position, such as when dropping an item of clothing.

    d4408   **Fine hand use, other specified**

    d4409   **Fine hand use, unspecified**

d445   Hand and arm use
Performing the coordinated actions required to move objects or to
manipulate them by using hands and arms, such as when turning door
handles or throwing or catching an object.

*Inclusions: pulling or pushing objects; reaching; turning or twisting the
hands or arms; throwing; catching*

Exclusion: fine hand use (d440)

d 4450   **Pulling**
Using fingers, hands and arms to bring an object towards
oneself, or to move it from place to place, such as when pulling
a door closed.

d 4451   **Pushing**
Using fingers, hands and arms to move something from
oneself, or to move it from place to place, such as when
pushing an animal away.

d 4452   **Reaching**
Using the hands and arms to extend outwards and touch and
grasp something, such as when reaching across a table or desk
for a book.

d 4453   **Turning or twisting the hands or arms**
Using fingers, hands and arms to rotate, turn or bend an
object, such as is required to use tools or utensils.

d 4454   **Throwing**
Using fingers, hands and arms to lift something and propel it
with some force through the air, such as when tossing a ball.

d 4455   **Catching**
Using fingers, hands and arms to grasp a moving object in
order to bring it to a stop and hold it, such as when catching a
ball.

d 4458   **Hand and arm use, other specified**

d 4459   **Hand and arm use, unspecified**

d449   Carrying, moving and handling objects, other specified and
unspecified

Walking and moving (d450-d469)

d 450   Walking
Moving along a surface on foot, step by step, so that one foot is always on the ground, such as when strolling, sauntering, walking forwards, backwards, or sideways.

Inclusions: walking short or long distances; walking on different surfaces; walking around obstacles

Exclusions: transferring oneself (d420); moving around (d455)

d 4500   Walking short distances
Walking for less than a kilometre, such as walking around rooms or hallways, within a building or for short distances outside.

d 4501   Walking long distances
Walking for more than a kilometre, such as across a village or town, between villages or across open areas.

d 4502   Walking on different surfaces
Walking on sloping, uneven, or moving surfaces, such as on grass, gravel or ice and snow, or walking aboard a ship, train or other vehicle.

d 4503   Walking around obstacles
Walking in ways required to avoid moving and immobile objects, people, animals, and vehicles, such as walking around a marketplace or shop, around or through traffic or other crowded areas.

d 4508   Walking, other specified

d 4509   Walking, unspecified

d 455   Moving around
Moving the whole body from one place to another by means other than walking, such as climbing over a rock or running down a street, skipping, scampering, jumping, somersaulting or running around obstacles.

Inclusions: crawling, climbing, running, jogging, jumping, and swimming

Exclusions: transferring oneself (d420); walking (d450)

d 4550   Crawling
Moving the whole body in a prone position from one place to another on hands, or hands and arms, and knees.

d 4551   Climbing
Moving the whole body upwards or downwards, over surfaces or objects, such as climbing steps, rocks, ladders or stairs, curbs or other objects.

d 4552   Running
Moving with quick steps so that both feet may be simultaneously off the ground.

d 4553   Jumping
Moving up off the ground by bending and extending the legs, such as jumping on one foot, hopping, skipping and jumping or diving into water.

d 4554   Swimming
Propelling the whole body through water by means of limb and body movements without taking support from the ground underneath.

d 4558   Moving around, other specified

d 4559   Moving around, unspecified

d 460   Moving around in different locations
Walking and moving around in various places and situations, such as walking between rooms in a house, within a building, or down the street of a town.

Inclusions: moving around within the home, crawling or climbing within the home; walking or moving within buildings other than the home, and outside the home and other buildings

d 4600   Moving around within the home
Walking and moving around in one's home, within a room, between rooms, and around the whole residence or living area.

Inclusions: moving from floor to floor, on an attached balcony, courtyard, porch or garden

d 4601   Moving around within buildings other than home
Walking and moving around within buildings other than one's
residence, such as moving around other people's homes, other
private buildings, community and private or public buildings
and enclosed areas.

*Inclusions: moving throughout all parts of buildings and
enclosed areas, between floors, inside, outside and around
buildings, both public and private*

d 4602   Moving around outside the home and other buildings
Walking and moving around close to or far from one's home
and other buildings, without the use of transportation, public
or private, such as walking for short or long distances around a
town or village.

*Inclusions: walking or moving down streets in the
neighbourhood, town, village or city; moving between cities and
further distances, without using transportation*

d 4608   Moving around in different locations, other specified

d 4609   Moving around in different locations, unspecified

d 465   Moving around using equipment
Moving the whole body from place to place, on any surface or space, by
using specific devices designed to facilitate moving or create other ways
of moving around, such as with skates, skis, or scuba equipment, or
moving down the street in a wheelchair or a walker.

*Exclusions: transferring oneself (d420); walking (d450); moving around
(d455); using transportation (d470); driving (d475)*

d 469   Walking and moving, other specified and unspecified

Moving around using transportation (d470-d489)

d 470   Using transportation
Using transportation to move around as a passenger, such as being
driven in a car or on a bus, rickshaw, jitney, animal-powered vehicle, or
private or public taxi, bus, train, tram, subway, boat or aircraft.

*Inclusions: using human-powered transportation; using private motorized
or public transportation*

Exclusions: moving around using equipment (d465); driving (d475)

d 4700   Using human-powered vehicles
Being transported as a passenger by a mode of transportation powered by one or more people, such as riding in a rickshaw or rowboat.

d 4701   Using private motorized transportation
Being transported as a passenger by private motorized vehicle over land, sea or air, such as by a taxi or privately owned aircraft or boat.

d 4702   Using public motorized transportation
Being transported as a passenger by a motorized vehicle over land, sea or air designed for public transportation, such as being a passenger on a bus, train, subway or aircraft.

d 4708   Using transportation, other specified

d 4709   Using transportation, unspecified

d 475   **Driving**
Being in control of and moving a vehicle or the animal that draws it, travelling under one's own direction or having at one's disposal any form of transportation, such as a car, bicycle, boat or animal-powered vehicle.

Inclusions: driving human-powered transportation, motorized vehicles, animal-powered vehicles

Exclusions: moving around using equipment (d465); using transportation (d470)

d 4750   Driving human-powered transportation
Driving a human-powered vehicle, such as a bicycle, tricycle, or rowboat.

d 4751   Driving motorized vehicles
Driving a vehicle with a motor, such as an automobile, motorcycle, motorboat or aircraft.

d 4752   Driving animal-powered vehicles
Driving a vehicle powered by an animal, such as a horse-drawn cart or carriage.

d 4758   Driving, other specified

d 4759   Driving, unspecified

d480   **Riding animals for transportation**
travelling on the back of an animal, such as a horse, ox, camel or
elephant

Exclusions: driving (d475); recreation and leisure (d920)

d489   **Moving around using transportation, other specified and
unspecified**

d498   **Mobility, other specified**

d499   **Mobility, unspecified**

Chapter 5
Self-care

This chapter is about caring for oneself, washing and drying oneself, caring for one's body and body parts, dressing, eating and drinking, and looking after one's health.

d510   **Washing oneself**

Washing and drying one's whole body, or body parts, using water and appropriate cleaning and drying materials or methods, such as bathing, showering, washing hands and feet, face and hair, and drying with a towel.

Inclusions: washing body parts, the whole body; and drying oneself

Exclusions: caring for body parts (d520); toileting (d530)

   d5100   **Washing body parts**

Applying water, soap and other substances to body parts, such as hands, face, feet, hair or nails, in order to clean them.

   d5101   **Washing whole body**

Applying water, soap and other substances to the whole body in order to clean oneself, such as taking a bath or shower.

   d5102   **Drying oneself**

Using a towel or other means for drying some part or parts of one's body, or the whole body, such as after washing.

   d5108   **Washing oneself, other specified**

   d5109   **Washing oneself, unspecified**

d520   **Caring for body parts**

Looking afer those parts of the body, such as skin, face, teeth, scalp, nails and genitals, that require more than washing and drying.

Inclusions: caring for skin, teeth, hair, finger and toe nails

Exclusions: washing oneself (d510); toileting (d530)

   d5200   **Caring for skin**

Looking after the texture and hydration of one's skin, such as by removing calluses or corns and using moisturizing lotions or cosmetics.

d 5201   **Caring for teeth**
Looking after dental hygiene, such as by brushing teeth, flossing, and taking care of a dental prosthesis or orthosis.

d 5202   **Caring for hair**
Looking after the hair on the head and face, such as by combing, styling, shaving, or trimming.

d 5203   **Caring for fingernails**
Cleaning, trimming or polishing the nails of the fingers.

d 5204   **Caring for toenails**
Cleaning, trimming or polishing the nails of the toes.

d 5208   **Caring for body parts, other specified**

d 5209   **Caring for body parts, unspecified**

d 530   **Toileting**
Planning and carrying out the elimination of human waste (menstruation, urination and defecation), and cleaning oneself afterwards.

Inclusions: regulating urination, defecation and menstrual care

Exclusions: washing oneself (d510); caring for body parts (d520)

d 5300   **Regulating urination**
Coordinating and managing urination, such as by indicating need, getting into the proper position, choosing and getting to an appropriate place for urination, manipulating clothing before and after urination, and cleaning oneself after urination.

d 5301   **Regulating defecation**
Coordinating and managing defecation such as by indicating need, getting into the proper position, choosing and getting to an appropriate place for defecation, manipulating clothing before and after defecation, and cleaning onself after defecation.

d 5302   **Menstrual care**
Coordinating, planning and caring for menstruation, such as by anticipating menstruation and using sanitary towels and napkins.

d 5308   **Toileting, other specified**

d 5309   Toileting, unspecified

d 540   **Dressing**
Carrying out the coordinated actions and tasks of putting on and taking off clothes and footwear in sequence and in keeping with climatic and social conditions, such as by putting on, adjusting and removing shirts, skirts, blouses, pants, undergarments, saris, kimono, tights, hats, gloves, coats, shoes, boots, sandals and slippers.

Inclusions: putting on or taking off clothes and footwear and choosing appropriate clothing

d 5400   **Putting on clothes**
Carrying out the coordinated tasks of putting clothes on various parts of the body, such as putting clothes on over the head, over the arms and shoulders, and on the lower and upper halves of the body; putting on gloves and headgear.

d 5401   **Taking off clothes**
Carrying out the coordinated tasks of taking clothes off various parts of the body, such as pulling clothes off and over the head, off the arms and shoulders, and off the lower and upper halves of the body; taking off gloves and headgear.

d 5402   **Putting on footwear**
Carrying out the coordinated tasks of putting on socks, stockings and footwear.

d 5403   **Taking off footwear**
Carrying out the coordinated tasks of taking off socks, stockings and footwear.

d 5404   **Choosing appropriate clothing**
Following implicit or explicit dress codes and conventions of one's society or culture and dressing in keeping with climatic conditions.

d 5408   Dressing, other specified

d 5409   Dressing, unspecified

d 550   **Eating**
Carrying out the coordinated tasks and actions of eating food that has been served, bringing it to the mouth and consuming it in culturally acceptable ways, cutting or breaking food into pieces, opening bottles and cans, using eating implements, having meals, feasting or dining.

Exclusion: drinking (d560)

d 560   **Drinking**
Taking hold of a drink, bringing it to the mouth, and consuming the drink in culturally acceptable ways, mixing, stirring and pouring liquids for drinking, opening bottles and cans, drinking through a straw or drinking running water such as from a tap or a spring; feeding from the breast.

Exclusion: eating (d550)

d 570   **Looking after one's health**
Ensuring physical comfort, health and physical and mental well-being, such as by maintaining a balanced diet, and an appropriate level of physical activity, keeping warm or cool, avoiding harms to health, following safe sex practices, including using condoms, getting immunizations and regular physical examinations.

Inclusions: ensuring one's physical comfort; managing diet and fitness; maintaining one's health

> **d 5700**   **Ensuring one's physical comfort**
> Caring for oneself by being aware that one needs to ensure, and ensuring, that one's body is in a comfortable position, that one is not feeling too hot or cold, and that one has adequate lighting.

> **d 5701**   **Managing diet and fitness**
> Caring for oneself by being aware of the need and by selecting and consuming nutritious foods and maintaining physical fitness.

> **d 5702**   **Maintaining one's health**
> Caring for oneself by being aware of the need and doing what is required to look after one's health, both to respond to risks to health and to prevent ill-health, such as by seeking professional assistance; following medical and other health advice; and avoiding risks to health such as physical injury, communicable diseases, drug-taking and sexually transmitted diseases.

> **d 5708**   **Looking after one's health, other specified**

> **d 5709**   **Looking after one's health, unspecified**

d 598   Self-care, other specified

d 599   Self-care, unspecified

Chapter 6
Domestic life

This chapter is about carrying out domestic and everyday actions and tasks. Areas of domestic life include acquiring a place to live, food, clothing and other necessities, household cleaning and repairing, caring for personal and other household objects, and assisting others.

Acquisition of necessities (d610-d629)

d610   **Acquiring a place to live**
Buying, renting, furnishing and arranging a house, apartment or other dwelling.

Inclusions: buying or renting a place to live and furnishing a place to live

Exclusions: acquisition of goods and services (d620); caring for household objects (d650)

> **d6100**   **Buying a place to live**
> Acquiring ownership of a house, apartment or other dwelling.

> **d6101**   **Renting a place to live**
> Acquiring the use of a house, apartment or other dwelling belonging to another in exchange for payment.

> **d6102**   **Furnishing a place to live**
> Equipping and arranging a living space with furniture, fixtures and other fittings and decorating rooms.

> **d6108**   **Acquiring a place to live, other specified**

> **d6109**   **Acquiring a place to live, unspecified**

d620   **Acquisition of goods and services**
Selecting, procuring and transporting all goods and services required for daily living, such as selecting, procuring, transporting and storing food, drink, clothing, cleaning materials, fuel, household items, utensils, cooking ware, domestic appliance and tools; procuring utilities and other household services.

Inclusions: shopping and gathering daily necessities

Exclusion: acquiring a place to live (d610)

d 6200   **Shopping**

Obtaining, in exchange for money, goods and services required for daily living (including instructing and supervising an intermediary to do the shopping), such as selecting food, drink, cleaning materials, household items or clothing in a shop or market; comparing quality and price of the items required, negotiating and paying for selected goods or services, and transporting goods.

d 6201   **Gathering daily necessities**

Obtaining, without exchange of money, goods and services required for daily living (including instructing and supervising an intermediate to gather daily necessities), such as by harvesting vegetables and fruits and getting water and fuel.

d 6208   **Acquisition of goods and services, other specified**

d 6209   **Acquisition of goods and services, unspecified**

d 629   Acquisition of necessities, other specified and unspecified

Household tasks (d630-d649)

d 630   Preparing meals

Planning, organizing, cooking and serving simple and complex meals for oneself and others, such as by making a menu, selecting edible food and drink, getting together ingredients for preparing meals, cooking with heat and preparing cold foods and drinks, and serving the food.

Inclusions: preparing simple and complex meals

Exclusions: eating (d550); drinking (d560); acquisition of goods and services (d620); doing housework (d640); caring for household objects (d650); caring for others (d660)

d 6300   **Preparing simple meals**

Organizing, cooking and serving meals with a small number of ingredients that require easy methods of preparation and serving, such as making a snack or small meal, and transforming food ingredients by cutting and stirring, boiling and heating food such as rice or potatoes.

d6301   Preparing complex meals

Planning, organizing, cooking and serving meals with a large number of ingredients that require complex methods of preparation and serving, such as planning a meal with several dishes, and transforming food ingredients by combined actions of peeling, slicing, mixing, kneading, stirring, presenting and serving food in a manner appropriate to the occasion and culture.

Exclusion: using household appliances (d6403)

d6308   Preparing meals, other specified

d6309   Preparing meals, unspecified

d640   Doing housework

Managing a household by cleaning the house, washing clothes, using household appliances, storing food and disposing of garbage, such as by sweeping, mopping, washing counters, walls and other surfaces; collecting and disposing of household garbage; tidying rooms, closets and drawers; collecting, washing, drying, folding and ironing clothes; cleaning footwear; using brooms, brushes and vacuum cleaners; using washing machines, driers and irons.

Inclusions: washing and drying clothes and garments; cleaning cooking area and utensils; cleaning living area; using household appliances, storing daily necessities and disposing of garbage

Exclusions: acquiring a place to live (d610); acquisition of goods and services (d620); preparing meals (d630); caring for household objects (d650); caring for others (d660)

d6400   Washing and drying clothes and garments

Washing clothes and garments by hand and hanging them out to dry in the air.

d6401   Cleaning cooking area and utensils

Cleaning up after cooking, such as by washing dishes, pans, pots and cooking utensils, and cleaning tables and floors around cooking and eating area.

d6402   Cleaning living area

Cleaning the living areas of the household, such as by tidying and dusting, sweeping, swabbing, mopping floors, cleaning windows and walls, cleaning bathrooms and toilets, cleaning household furnishings.

d 6403   Using household appliances
Using all kinds of household appliances, such as washing machines, driers, irons, vacuum cleaners and dishwashers.

d 6404   Storing daily necessities
Storing food, drinks, clothes and other household goods required for daily living; preparing food for conservation by canning, salting or refrigerating, keeping food fresh and out of the reach of animals.

d 6405   Disposing of garbage
Disposing of household garbage such as by collecting trash and rubbish around the house, preparing garbage for disposal, using garbage disposal appliances; burning garbage.

d 6408   Doing housework, other specified

d 6409   Doing housework, unspecified

d 649   Household tasks, other specified and unspecified

Caring for household objects and assisting others (d650-d669)

d 650   Caring for household objects
Maintaining and repairing household and other personal objects, including house and contents, clothes, vehicles and assistive devices, and caring for plants and animals, such as painting or wallpapering rooms, fixing furniture, repairing plumbing, ensuring the proper working order of vehicles, watering plants, grooming and feeding pets and domestic animals.

Inclusions: making and repairing clothes; maintaining dwelling, furnishings and domestic appliances; maintaining vehicles; maintaining assistive devices; taking care of plants (indoor and outdoor) and animals

Exclusions: acquiring a place to live (d610); acquisition of goods and services (d620); doing housework (d640); caring for others (d660); remunerative employment (d850)

d 6500   Making and repairing clothes
Making and repairing clothes, such as by sewing, producing or mending clothes; reattaching buttons and fasteners; ironing clothes, fixing and polishing footwear.

Exclusion: using household appliances (d6403)

d 6501   Maintaining dwelling and furnishings
Repairing and taking care of dwelling, its exterior, interior and contents, such as by painting, repairing fixtures and furniture, and using required tools for repair work.

d 6502   Maintaining domestic appliances
Repairing and taking care of all domestic appliances for cooking, cleaning and repairing, such as by oiling and repairing tools and maintaining the washing machine.

d 6503   Maintaining vehicles
Repairing and taking care of motorized and non-motorized vehicles for personal use, including bicycles, carts, automobiles and boats.

d 6504   Maintaining assistive devices
Repairing and taking care of assistive devices, such as prostheses, orthoses and specialized tools and aids for housekeeping and personal care; maintaining and repairing aids for personal mobility such as canes, walkers, wheelchairs and scooters; and maintaining communication and recreational aids.

d 6505   Taking care of plants, indoors and outdoors
Taking care of plants inside and outside the house, such as by planting, watering and fertilizing plants; gardening and growing foods for personal use.

d 6506   Taking care of animals
Taking care of domestic animals and pets, such as by feeding, cleaning, grooming and exercising pets; watching over the health of animals or pets; planning for the care of animals or pets in one's absence.

d 6508   Caring for household objects, specified

d 6509   Caring for household objects, unspecified

d 660   **Assisting others**
Assisting household members and others with their learning, communicating, self-care, movement, within the house or outside; being concerned about the well-being of household members and others.

Inclusions: assisting others with self-care, movement, communication, interpersonal relations, nutrition and health maintenance

Exclusion: remunerative employment (d850)

d 6600 Assisting others with self-care

Assisting household members and others in performing self-care, including helping others with eating, bathing and dressing; taking care of children or members of the household who are sick or have difficulties with basic self-care; helping others with their toileting.

d 6601 Assisting others in movement

Assisting household members and others in movements and in moving outside the home, such as in the neighbourhood or city, to or from school, place of employment or other destination.

d 6602 Assisting others in communication

Assisting household members and others with their communication, such as by helping with speaking, writing or reading.

d 6603 Assisting others in interpersonal relations

Assisting household members and others with their interpersonal interactions, such as by helping them to initiate, maintain or terminate relationships.

d 6604 Assisting others in nutrition

Assisting household members and others with their nutrition, such as by helping them to prepare and eat meals.

d 6605 Assisting others in health maintenance

Assisting household members and others with formal and informal health care, such as by ensuring that a child gets regular medical check-ups, or that an elderly relative takes required medication.

d 6608 Assisting others, other specified

d 6609 Assisting others, unspecified

d 669 Caring for household objects and assisting others, other specified and unspecified

d 698 Domestic life, other specified

d 699 Domestic life, unspecified

Chapter 7

Interpersonal interactions and relationships

This chapter is about carrying out the actions and tasks required for basic and complex interactions with people (strangers, friends, relatives, family members and lovers) in a contextually and socially appropriate manner.

General interpersonal interactions (d710-d729)

d710 **Basic interpersonal interactions**
Interacting with people in a contextually and socially appropriate manner, such as by showing consideration and esteem when appropriate, or responding to the feelings of others.

Inclusions: showing respect, warmth, appreciation, and tolerance in relationships; responding to criticism and social cues in relationships; and using appropriate physical contact in relationships

d7100 **Respect and warmth in relationships**
Showing and responding to consideration and esteem, in a contextually and socially appropriate manner.

d7101 **Appreciation in relationships**
Showing and responding to satisfaction and gratitude, in a contextually and socially appropriate manner.

d7102 **Tolerance in relationships**
Showing and responding to understanding and acceptance of behaviour, in a contextually and socially appropriate manner.

d7103 **Criticism in relationships**
Providing and responding to implicit and explicit differences of opinion or disagreement, in a contextually and socially appropriate manner.

d7104 **Social cues in relationships**
Giving and reacting appropriately to signs and hints that occur in social interactions.

d7105 **Physical contact in relationships**
Making and responding to bodily contact with others, in a contextually and socially appropriate manner.

159

d 7108 Basic interpersonal interactions, other specified

d 7109 Basic interpersonal interactions, unspecified

d 720 Complex interpersonal interactions
Maintaining and managing interactions with other people, in a contextually and socially appropriate manner, such as by regulating emotions and impulses, controlling verbal and physical aggression, acting independently in social interactions, and acting in accordance with social rules and conventions.

Inclusions: forming and terminating relationships; regulating behaviours within interactions; interacting according to social rules; and maintaining social space

d 7200 Forming relationships
Beginning and maintaining interactions with others for a short or long period of time, in a contextually and socially appropriate manner, such as by introducing oneself, finding and establishing friendships and professional relationships, starting a relationship that may become permanent, romantic or intimate.

d 7201 Terminating relationships
Bringing interactions to a close in a contextually and socially appropriate manner, such as by ending temporary relationships at the end of a visit, ending long-term relationships with friends when moving to a new town or ending relationships with work colleagues, professional colleagues and service providers, and ending romantic or intimate relationships.

d 7202 Regulating behaviours within interactions
Regulating emotions and impulses, verbal aggression and physical aggression in interactions with others, in a contextually and socially appropriate manner.

d 7203 Interacting according to social rules
Acting independently in social interactions and complying with social conventions governing one's role, position or other social status in interactions with others.

d 7204 Maintaining social space
Being aware of and maintaining a distance between oneself and others that is contextually, socially and culturally appropriate.

d 7208 Complex interpersonal interactions, other specified

d7209   Complex interpersonal interactions, unspecified

d729   General interpersonal interactions, other specified and unspecified

Particular interpersonal relationships (d730-d779)

d730   Relating with strangers
Engaging in temporary contacts and links with strangers for specific purposes, such as when asking for directions or making a purchase.

d740   Formal relationships
Creating and maintaining specific relationships in formal settings, such as with employers, professionals or service providers.

Inclusions: relating with persons in authority, with subordinates and with equals

d7400   Relating with persons in authority
Creating and maintaining formal relations with people in positions of power or of a higher rank or prestige relative to one's own social position, such as an employer.

d7401   Relating with subordinates
Creating and maintaining formal relations with people in positions of lower rank or prestige relative to one's own social position, such as an employee or servant.

d7402   Relating with equals
Creating and maintaining formal relations with people in the same position of authority, rank or prestige relative to one's own social position.

d7408   Formal relationships, other specified

d7409   Formal relationships, other unspecified

d750   Informal social relationships
Entering into relationships with others, such as casual relationships with people living in the same community or residence, or with co-workers, students, playmates or people with similar backgrounds or professions.

Inclusions: informal relationships with friends, neighbours, acquaintances, co-inhabitants and peers

d 7500   **Informal relationships with friends**
Creating and maintaining friendship relationships that are characterized by mutual esteem and common interests.

d 7501   **Informal relationships with neighbours**
Creating and maintaining informal relationships with people who live in nearby dwellings or living areas.

d 7502   **Informal relationships with acquaintances**
Creating and maintaining informal relationships with people whom one knows but who are not close friends.

d 7503   **Informal relationships with co-inhabitants**
Creating and maintaining informal relationships with people who are co-inhabitants of a house or other dwelling, privately or publicly run, for any purpose.

d 7504   **Informal relationships with peers**
Creating and maintaining informal relationships with people who share the same age, interest or other common feature.

d 7508   **Informal social relationships, other specified**

d 7509   **Informal social relationships, unspecified**

d 760   **Family relationships**
Creating and maintaining kinship relationships, such as with members of the nuclear family, extended family, foster and adopted family and step-relationships, more distant relationships such as second cousins, or legal guardians.

Inclusions: parent-child and child-parent relationships, sibling and extended family relationships

d 7600   **Parent-child relationships**
Becoming and being a parent, both natural and adoptive, such as by having a child and relating to it as a parent or creating and maintaining a parental relationship with an adoptive child, and providing physical, intellectual and emotional nurture to one's natural or adoptive child.

d 7601   **Child-parent relationships**
Creating and maintaining relationships with one's parent, such as a young child obeying his or her parents or an adult child taking care of his or her elderly parents.

d7602   Sibling relationships
Creating and maintaining a brotherly or sisterly relationship with a person who shares one or both parents by birth, adoption or marriage.

d7603   Extended family relationships
Creating and maintaining a family relationship with members of one's extended family, such as with cousins, aunts and uncles and grandparents.

d7608   Family relationships, other specified

d7609   Family relationships, unspecified

d770   Intimate relationships
Creating and maintaining close or romantic relationships between individuals, such as husband and wife, lovers or sexual partners.

Inclusions: romantic, spousal and sexual relationships

d7700   Romantic relationships
Creating and maintaining a relationship based on emotional and physical attraction, potentially leading to long-term intimate relationships.

d7701   Spousal relationships
Creating and maintaining an intimate relationship of a legal nature with another person, such as in a legal marriage, including becoming and being a legally married wife or husband or an unmarried spouse.

d7702   Sexual relationships
Creating and maintaining a relationship of a sexual nature, with a spouse or other partner.

d7708   Intimate relationships, other specified

d7709   Intimate relationships, unspecified

d779   Particular interpersonal relationships, other specified and unspecified

d798   Interpersonal interactions and relationships, other specified

d799   Interpersonal interactions and relationships, unspecified

Chapter 8
Major life areas

This chapter is about carrying out the tasks and actions required to engage in education, work and employment and to conduct economic transactions.

Education (d810-d839)

d810 **Informal education**

Learning at home or in some other non-institutional setting, such as learning crafts and other skills from parents or family members, or home schooling.

d815 **Preschool education**

Learning at an initial level of organized instruction, designed primarily to introduce a child to the school-type environment and prepare it for compulsory education, such as by acquiring skills in a day-care or similar setting as preparation for advancement to school.

d820 **School education**

Gaining admission to school, Education, engaging in all school-related responsibilities and privileges, and learning the course material, subjects and other curriculum requirements in a primary or secondary education programme, including attending school regularly, working cooperatively with other students, taking direction from teachers, organizing, studying and completing assigned tasks and projects, and advancing to other stages of education.

d825 **Vocational training**

Engaging in all activities of a vocational programme and learning the curriculum material in preparation for employment in a trade, job or profession.

d830 **Higher education**

Engaging in the activities of advanced educational programmes in universities, colleges and professional schools and learning all aspects of the curriculum required for degrees, diplomas, certificates and other accreditations, such as completing a university bachelor's or master's course of study, medical school or other professional school.

d839 **Education, other specified and unspecified**

Work and employment (d840-d859)

d840   **Apprenticeship (work preparation)**
Engaging in programmes related to preparation for employment, such as performing the tasks required of an apprenticeship, internship, articling and in-service training.

Exclusion: vocational training (d825)

d845   **Acquiring, keeping and terminating a job**
Seeking, finding and choosing employment, being hired and accepting employment, maintaining and advancing through a job, trade, occupation or profession, and leaving a job in an appropriate manner.

Inclusions: seeking employment; preparing a resume or curriculum vitae; contacting employers and preparing interviews; maintaining a job; monitoring one's own work performance; giving notice; and terminating a job

     d8450   **Seeking employment**
Locating and choosing a job, in a trade, profession or other form of employment, and performing the required tasks to get hired, such as showing up at the place of employment or participating in a job interview.

     d8451   **Maintaining a job**
Performing job-related tasks to keep an occupation, trade, profession or other form of employment, and obtaining promotion and other advancements in employment.

     d8452   **Terminating a job**
Leaving or quitting a job in the appropriate manner.

     d8458   **Acquiring, keeping and terminating a job, other specified**

     d8459   **Acquiring, keeping and terminating a job, unspecified**

d850   **Remunerative employment**
Engaging in all aspects of work, as an occupation, trade, profession or other form of employment, for payment, as an employee, full or part time, or self-employed, such as seeking employment and getting a job, doing the required tasks of the job, attending work on time as required, supervising other workers or being supervised, and performing required tasks alone or in groups.

Inclusions: self-employment, part-time and full-time employment

d 8500   Self-employment
Engaging in remunerative work sought or generated by the
individual, or contracted from others without a formal
employment relationship, such as migratory agricultural work,
working as a free-lance writer or consultant, short-term
contract work, working as an artist or crafts person, owning
and running a shop or other business.

Exclusions: part-time and full-time employment (d8501, d8502)

d 8501   Part-time employment
Engaging in all aspects of work for payment on a part-time
basis, as an employee, such as seeking employment and getting
a job, doing the tasks required of the job, attending work on
time as required, supervising other workers or being
supervised, and performing required tasks alone or in groups.

d 8502   Full-time employment
Engaging in all aspects of work for payment on a full-time
basis, as an employee, such as seeking employment and getting
a job, doing the required tasks of the job, attending work on
time as required, supervising other workers or being
supervised, and performing required tasks alone or in groups.

d 8508   Remunerative employment, other specified

d 8509   Remunerative employment, unspecified

d 855   Non-remunerative employment
Engaging in all aspects of work in which pay is not provided, full-time or
part-time, including organized work activities, doing the required tasks
of the job, attending work on time as required, supervising other
workers or being supervised, and performing required tasks alone or in
groups, such as volunteer work, charity work, working for a community
or religious group without remuneration, working around the home
without remuneration.

Exclusion: Chapter 6 Domestic Life

d 859   Work and employment, other specified and unspecified

Economic life (d860-d879)

d 860   Basic economic transactions
Engaging in any form of simple economic transaction, such as using
money to purchase food or bartering, exchanging goods or services; or
saving money.

d 865 **Complex economic transactions**
Engaging in any form of complex economic transaction that involves
the exchange of capital or property, and the creation of profit or
economic value, such as buying a business, factory, or equipment,
maintaining a bank account, or trading in commodities.

d 870 **Economic self-sufficiency**
Having command over economic resources, from private or public
sources, in order to ensure economic security for present and future
needs.

Inclusions: personal economic resources and public economic entitlements

d 8700 **Personal economic resources**
Having command over personal or private economic
resources, in order to ensure economic security for present and
future needs.

d 8701 **Public economic entitlements**
Having command over public economic resources, in order to
ensure economic security for present and future needs.

d 8708 **Economic self-sufficiency, other specified**

d 8709 **Economic self-sufficiency, unspecified**

d 879 **Economic life, other specified and unspecified**

d 898 **Major life areas, other specified**

d 899 **Major life areas, unspecified**

Chapter 9
Community, social and civic life

This chapter is about the actions and tasks required to engage in organized social life outside the family, in community, social and civic areas of life.

d910 **Community life**

Engaging in all aspects of community social life, such as engaging in charitable organizations, service clubs or professional social organizations.

Inclusions: informal and formal associations; ceremonies

Exclusions: non-remunerative employment (d855); recreation and leisure (d920); religion and spirituality (d930); political life and citizenship (d950)

d9100 **Informal associations**

Engaging in social or community associations organized by people with common interests, such as local social clubs or ethnic groups.

d9101 **Formal associations**

Engaging in professional or other exclusive social groups, such as associations of lawyers, physicians or academics.

d9102 **Ceremonies**

Engaging in non-religious rites or social ceremonies, such as marriages, funerals or initiation ceremonies.

d9108 **Community life, other specified**

d9109 **Community life, unspecified**

d920 **Recreation and leisure**

Engaging in any form of play, recreational or leisure activity, such as informal or organized play and sports, programmes of physical fitness, relaxation, amusement or diversion, going to art galleries, museums, cinemas or theatres; engaging in crafts or hobbies, reading for enjoyment, playing musical instruments; sightseeing, tourism and travelling for pleasure.

Inclusions: play, sports, arts and culture, crafts, hobbies and socializing

Exclusions: riding animals for transportation (d480); remunerative and non-remunerative work (d850 and d855); religion and spirituality (d930); political life and citizenship (d950)

d 9200   Play
Engaging in games with rules or unstructured or unorganized games and spontaneous recreation, such as playing chess or cards or children's play.

d 9201   Sports
Engaging in competitive and informal or formally organized games or athletic events, performed alone or in a group, such as bowling, gymnastics or soccer.

d 9202   Arts and culture
Engaging in, or appreciating, fine arts or cultural events, such as going to the theatre, cinema, museum or art gallery, or acting in a play, reading for enjoyment or playing a musical instrument.

d 9203   Crafts
Engaging in handicrafts, such as pottery or knitting.

d 9204   Hobbies
Engaging in pastimes such as collecting stamps, coins or antiques.

d 9205   Socializing
Engaging in informal or casual gatherings with others, such as visiting friends or relatives or meeting informally in public places.

d 9208   Recreation and leisure, other specified

d 9209   Recreation and leisure, unspecified

d930   **Religion and spirituality**
Engaging in religious or spiritual activities, organizations and practices for self-fulfilment, finding meaning, religious or spiritual value and establishing connection with a divine power, such as is involved in attending a church, temple, mosque or synagogue, praying or chanting for a religious purpose, and spiritual contemplation.

Inclusions: organized religion and spirituality

d 9300   Organized religion
Engaging in organized religious ceremonies, activities and events.

d 9301   **Spirituality**
Engaging in spiritual activities or events, outside an organized religion.

d 9308   **Religion and spirituality, other specified**

d 9309   **Religion and spirituality, unspecified**

d 940   Human rights
Enjoying all nationally and internationally recognized rights that are accorded to people by virtue of their humanity alone, such as human rights as recognized by the United Nations Universal Declaration of Human Rights (1948) and the United Nations Standard Rules for the Equalization of Opportunities for Persons with Disabilities (1993); the right to self-determination or autonomy; and the right to control over one's destiny.

Exclusion: political life and citizenship (d950)

d 950   Political life and citizenship
Engaging in the social, political and governmental life of a citizen, having legal status as a citizen and enjoying the rights, protections, privileges and duties associated with that role, such as the right to vote and run for political office, to form political associations; enjoying the rights and freedoms associated with citizenship (e.g. the rights of freedom of speech, association, religion, protection against unreasonable search and seizure, the right to counsel, to a trial and other legal rights and protection against discrimination); having legal standing as a citizen.

Exclusion: human rights (d940)

d 998   Community, social and civic life, other specified

d 999   Community, social and civic life, unspecified

ENVIRONMENTAL FACTORS

Definition: *Environmental factors make up the physical, social and attitudinal environment in which people live and conduct their lives.*

Coding environmental factors

Environmental Factors is a component of Part 2 (Contextual factors) of the classification. These factors must be considered for each component of functioning and coded accordingly (see Annex 2).

Environmental factors are to be coded from the perspective of the person whose situation is being described. For example, kerb cuts without textured paving may be coded as a facilitator for a wheelchair user but as a barrier for a blind person.

The first qualifier indicates the extent to which a factor is a facilitator or a barrier. There are several reasons why an environmental factor may be a facilitator or a barrier, and to what extent. For facilitators, the coder should keep in mind issues such as the accessibility of a resource, and whether access is dependable or variable, of good or poor quality, and so on. In the case of barriers, it might be relevant how often a factor hinders the person, whether the hindrance is great or small, or avoidable or not. It should also be kept in mind that an environmental factor can be a barrier either because of its presence (for example, negative attitudes towards people with disabilities) or its absence (for example, the unavailability of a needed service). The effects that environmental factors have on the lives of people with health conditions are varied and complex, and it is hoped that future research will lead to better understanding of this interaction and, possibly, show the usefulness of a second qualifier for these factors.

In some instances, a diverse collection of environmental factors is summarized with a single term, such as poverty, development, rural or urban setting or social capital. These summary terms are not themselves found in the classification. Rather, the coder should separate the constituent factors and code these. Once again, further research is required to determine whether there are clear and consistent sets of environmental factors that make up each of these summary terms.

First qualifier

The following is the negative and positive scale for the extent to which an environmental factor acts as a barrier or a facilitator. A point or separator alone denotes a barrier, and the + sign denotes a facilitator, as indicated below:

xxx.0 NO barrier	(none, absent, negligible,…)	0-4%
xxx.1 MILD barrier	(slight, low,…)	5-24%
xxx.2 MODERATE barrier	(medium, fair,...)	25-49%
xxx.3 SEVERE barrier	(high, extreme, …)	50-95%
xxx.4 COMPLETE barrier	(total,…)	96-100%
xxx+0 NO facilitator	(none, absent, negligible,…)	0-4%
xxx+1 MILD facilitator	(slight, low,…)	5-24%
xxx+2 MODERATE facilitator	(medium, fair,...)	25-49%
xxx+3 SUBSTANTIAL facilitator	(high, extreme, …)	50-95%
xxx+4 COMPLETE facilitator	(total,…)	96-100%

xxx.8 barrier, not specified
xxx+8 facilitator, not specified
xxx.9 not applicable

Broad ranges of percentages are provided for those cases in which calibrated assessment instruments or other standards are available to quantify the extent of the barrier or facilitator in the environment. For example, when "no barrier" or a "complete barrier" is coded, this scaling has a margin of error of up to 5%. A "moderate barrier" is defined as up to half of the scale of a total barrier. The percentages are to be calibrated in different domains with reference to population standards as percentiles. For this quantification to be used in a uniform manner, assessment procedures have to be developed through research.

Second qualifier: To be developed.

Chapter 1
Products and technology

This chapter is about the natural or human-made products or systems of products, equipment and technology in an individual's immediate environment that are gathered, created, produced or manufactured. The ISO 9999 classification of technical aids defines these as "any product, instrument, equipment or technical system used by a disabled person, especially produced or generally available, preventing, compensating, monitoring, relieving or neutralizing" disability. It is recognized that any product or technology can be assistive. (See ISO 9999: Technical aids for disabled persons - Classification (second version); ISO/TC 173/SC 2; ISO/DIS 9999 (rev.).) For the purposes of this classification of environmental factors, however, assistive products and technology are defined more narrowly as any product, instrument, equipment or technology adapted or specially designed for improving the functioning of a disabled person.

e110 **Products or substances for personal consumption**
Any natural or human-made object or substance gathered, processed or manufactured for ingestion.

Inclusions: food and drugs

    e1100 **Food**
Any natural or human-made object or substance gathered, processed or manufactured to be eaten, such as raw, processed and prepared food and liquids of different consistencies, herbs and minerals (vitamin and other supplements).

    e1101 **Drugs**
Any natural or human-made object or substance gathered, processed or manufactured for medicinal purposes, such as allopathic and naturopathic medication.

    e1108 **Products or substances for personal consumption, other specified**

    e1109 **Products or substances for personal consumption, unspecified**

e115 **Products and technology for personal use in daily living**
Equipment, products and technologies used by people in daily activities, including those adapted or specially designed, located in, on or near the person using them.

Inclusions: general and assistive products and technology for personal use

e1150   **General products and technology for personal use in daily living**
Equipment, products and technologies used by people in daily activities, such as clothes, textiles, furniture, appliances, cleaning products and tools, not adapted or specially designed.

e1151   **Assistive products and technology for personal use in daily living**
Adapted or specially designed equipment, products and technologies that assist people in daily living, such as prosthetic and orthotic devices, neural prostheses (e.g. functional stimulation devices that control bowels, bladder, breathing and heart rate), and environmental control units aimed at facilitating individuals' control over their indoor setting (scanners, remote control systems, voice-controlled systems, timer switches).

e1158   **Products and technology for personal use in daily living, other specified**

e1159   **Products and technology for personal use in daily living, unspecified**

e120   **Products and technology for personal indoor and outdoor mobility and transportation**
Equipment, products and technologies used by people in activities of moving inside and outside buildings, including those adapted or specially designed, located in, on or near the person using them.

Inclusions: general and assistive products and technology for personal indoor and outdoor mobility and transportation

e1200   **General products and technology for personal indoor and outdoor mobility and transportation**
Equipment, products and technologies used by people in activities of moving inside and outside buildings, such as motorized and non-motorized vehicles used for the transportation of people over ground, water and air (e.g. buses, cars, vans, other motor-powered vehicles and animal-powered transporters), not adapted or specially designed.

e1201   **Assistive products and technology for personal indoor and outdoor mobility and transportation**
Adapted or specially designed equipment, products and technologies that assist people to move inside and outside buildings, such as walking devices, special cars and vans, adaptations to vehicles, wheelchairs, scooters and transfer devices.

    e1208   **Products and technology for personal indoor and outdoor mobility and transportation, other specified**

    e1209   **Products and technology for personal indoor and outdoor mobility and transportation, unspecified**

e125   **Products and technology for communication**
Equipment, products and technologies used by people in activities of sending and receiving information, including those adapted or specially designed, located in, on or near the person using them.

Inclusions: general and assistive products and technology for communication

    e1250   **General products and technology for communication**
Equipment, products and technologies used by people in activities of sending and receiving information, such as optical and auditory devices, audio recorders and receivers, television and video equipment, telephone devices, sound transmission systems and face-to-face communication devices, not adapted or specially designed.

    e1251   **Assistive products and technology for communication**
Adapted or specially designed equipment, products and technologies that assist people to send and receive information, such as specialized vision devices, electro-optical devices, specialized writing devices, drawing or handwriting devices, signalling systems and special computer software and hardware, cochlear implants, hearing aids, FM auditory trainers, voice prostheses, communication boards, glasses and contact lenses.

    e1258   **Products and technology for communication, other specified**

    e1259   **Products and technology for communication, unspecified**

e130   **Products and technology for education**
Equipment, products, processes, methods and technology used for acquisition of knowledge, expertise or skill, including those adapted or specially designed.

Inclusions: general and assistive products and technology for education

e 1300   General products and technology for education
Equipment, products, processes, methods and technology used
for acquisition of knowledge, expertise or skill at any level,
such as books, manuals, educational toys, computer hardware
or software, not adapted or specially designed.

e 1301   Assistive products and technology for education
Adapted and specially designed equipment, products,
processes, methods and technology used for acquisition of
knowledge, expertise or skill, such as specialized computer
technology.

e 1308   Products and technology for education, other specified

e 1309   Products and technology for education, unspecified

e 135   Products and technology for employment
Equipment, products and technology used for employment to facilitate
work activities.

Inclusions: general and assistive products and technology for employment

e 1350   General products and technology for employment
Equipment, products and technology used for employment to
facilitate work activities, such as tools, machines and office
equipment, not adapted or specially designed.

e 1351   Assistive products and technology for employment
Adapted or specially designed equipment, products and
technology used for employment to facilitate work activities,
such as adjustable tables, desks and filing cabinets; remote
control entry and exit of office doors; computer hardware,
software, accessories and environmental control units aimed at
facilitating an individual's conduct of work-related tasks and
aimed at control of the work environment (e.g. scanners,
remote control systems, voice-controlled systems and timer
switches).

e 1358   Products and technology for employment, other specified

e 1359   Products and technology for employment, unspecified

e140   **Products and technology for culture, recreation and sport**
Equipment, products and technology used for the conduct and
enhancement of cultural, recreational and sporting activities, including
those adapted or specially designed.

*Inclusions: general and assistive products and technology for culture,
recreation and sport*

> **e1400**   **General products and technology for culture, recreation and**
> **sport**
> Equipment, products and technology used for the conduct and
> enhancement of cultural, recreational and sporting activities,
> such as toys, skis, tennis balls and musical instruments, not
> adapted or specially designed.

> **e1401**   **Assistive products and technology for culture, recreation**
> **and sport**
> Adapted or specially designed equipment, products and
> technology used for the conduct and enhancement of cultural,
> recreational and sporting activities, such as modified mobility
> devices for sports, adaptations for musical and other artistic
> performance.

> **e1408**   **Products and technology for culture, recreation and sport,**
> **other specified**

> **e1409**   **Products and technology for culture, recreation and sport,**
> **unspecified**

e145   **Products and technology for the practice of religion and spirituality**
Products and technology, unique or mass-produced, that are given or
take on a symbolic meaning in the context of the practice of religion or
spirituality, including those adapted or specially designed.

*Inclusions: general and assistive products and technology for the practice
of religion and spirituality*

> **e1450**   **General products and technology for the practice of religion**
> **or spirituality**
> Products and technology, unique or mass-produced, that are
> given or take on a symbolic meaning in the context of the
> practice of religion or spirituality, such as spirit houses,
> maypoles, headdresses, masks, crucifixes, menorahs and
> prayer mats, not adapted or specially designed.

e 1451   **Assistive products and technology for the practice of religion or spirituality**
Adapted or specially designed products and technology that are given, or take on a symbolic meaning in the context of the practice of religion or spirituality, such as Braille religious books, Braille tarot cards, and special protection for wheelchair wheels when entering temples.

e 1458   **Products and technology for the practice of religion or spirituality, other specified**

e 1459   **Products and technology for the practice of religion or spirituality, unspecified**

e 150   **Design, construction and building products and technology of buildings for public use**
Products and technology that constitute an individual's indoor and outdoor human-made environment that is planned, designed and constructed for public use, including those adapted or specially designed.

Inclusions: design, construction and building products and technology of entrances and exits, facilities and routing

e 1500   **Design, construction and building products and technology for entering and exiting buildings for public use**
Products and technology of entry and exit from the human-made environment that is planned, designed and constructed for public use, such as design, building and construction of entries and exits to buildings for public use (e.g. workplaces, shops and theatres), public buildings, portable and stationary ramps, power-assisted doors, lever door handles and level door thresholds.

e 1501   **Design, construction and building products and technology for gaining access to facilities inside buildings for public use**
Products and technology of indoor facilities in design, building and construction for public use, such as washroom facilities, telephones, audio loops, lifts or elevators, escalators, thermostats (for temperature regulation) and dispersed accessible seating in auditoriums or stadiums.

e 1502   **Design, construction and building products and technology for way finding, path routing and designation of locations in buildings for public use**
Indoor and outdoor products and technology in design, building and construction for public use to assist people to find their way inside and immediately outside buildings and locate the places they want to go to, such as signage, in Braille or writing, size of corridors, floor surfaces, accessible kiosks and other forms of directories.

e 1508   **Design, construction and building products and technology of buildings for public use, other specified**

e 1509   **Design, construction and building products and technology of buildings for public use, unspecified**

e 155   **Design, construction and building products and technology of buildings for private use**
Products and technology that constitute an individual's indoor and outdoor human-made environment that is planned, designed and constructed for private use, including those adapted or specially designed.

Inclusions: design, construction and building products and technology of entrances and exits, facilities and routing

e 1550   **Design, construction and building products and technology for entering and exiting of buildings for private use**
Products and technology of entry and exit from the human-made environment that is planned, designed and constructed for private use, such as entries and exits to private homes, portable and stationary ramps, power-assisted doors, lever door handles and level door thresholds.

e 1551   **Design, construction and building products and technology for gaining access to facilities in buildings for private use**
Products and technology related to design, building and construction inside buildings for private use, such as washroom facilities, telephones, audio loops, kitchen cabinets, appliances and electronic controls in private homes.

e 1552   **Design, construction and building products and technology for way finding, path routing and designation of locations in buildings for private use**

Indoor and outdoor products and technology in the design, building and construction of path routing, for private use, to assist people to find their way inside and immediately outside buildings and locate the places they want to go to, such as signage, in Braille or writing, size of corridors and floor surfaces.

e 1558   **Design, construction and building products and technology of buildings for private use, other specified**

e 1559   **Design, construction and building products and technology of buildings for private use, unspecified**

e160   **Products and technology of land development**

Products and technology of land areas, as they affect an individual's outdoor environment through the implementation of land use policies, design, planning and development of space, including those adapted or specially designed.

Inclusions: products and technology of land areas that have been organized by the implementation of land use policies, such as rural areas, suburban areas, urban areas, parks, conservation areas and wildlife reserves

e 1600   **Products and technology of rural land development**

Products and technology in rural land areas, as they affect an individual's outdoor environment through the implementation of rural land use policies, design, planning and development of space, such as farm lands, pathways and signposting.

e 1601   **Products and technology of suburban land development**

Products and technology in suburban land areas, as they affect an individual`s outdoor environment through the implementation of suburban land use policies, design, planning and development of space, such as kerb cuts, pathways, signposting and street lighting.

e 1602   **Products and technology of urban land development**

Products and technology in urban land areas as they affect an individual`s outdoor environment through the implementation of urban land use policies, design, planning and development of space, such as kerb cuts, ramps, signposting and street lighting.

e 1603   **Products and technology of parks, conservation and wildlife areas**
Products and technology in land areas making up parks, conservation and wildlife areas, as they affect an individual`s outdoor environment through the implementation of land use policies and design, planning and development of space, such as park signage and wildlife trails.

e 1608   **Products and technology of land development, other specified**

e 1609   **Products and technology of land development, unspecified**

e 165   **Assets**
Products or objects of economic exchange such as money, goods, property and other valuables that an individual owns or of which he or she has rights of use.

Inclusions: tangible and intangible products and goods, financial assets

e 1650   **Financial assets**
Products, such as money and other financial instruments, which serve as a medium of exchange for labour, capital goods and services.

e 1651   **Tangible assets**
Products or objects, such as houses and land, clothing, food and technical goods, which serve as a medium of exchange for labour, capital goods and services.

e 1652   **Intangible assets**
Products, such as intellectual property, knowledge and skills, which serve as a medium of exchange for labour, capital goods and services.

e 1658   **Assets, other specified**

e 1659   **Assets, unspecified**

e 198   **Products and technology, other specified**

e 199   **Products and technology, unspecified**

Chapter 2
Natural environment and human-made changes to environment

This chapter is about animate and inanimate elements of the natural or physical environment, and components of that environment that have been modified by people, as well as characteristics of human populations within that environment.

e210 Physical geography
Features of land forms and bodies of water.

Inclusions: features of geography included within orography (relief, quality and expanse of land and land forms, including altitude) and hydrography (bodies of water such as lakes, rivers, sea)

e2100 **Land forms**
Features of land forms, such as mountains, hills, valleys and plains.

e2101 **Bodies of water**
Features of bodies of water, such as lakes, dams, rivers and streams.

e2108 **Physical geography, other specified**

e2109 **Physical geography, unspecified**

e215 Population
Groups of people living in a given environment who share the same pattern of environmental adaptation.

Inclusions: demographic change; population density

e2150 **Demographic change**
Changes occurring within groups of people, such as the composition and variation in the total number of individuals in an area caused by birth, death, ageing of a population and migration.

e2151 **Population density**
Number of people per unit of land area, including features such as high and low density.

e2158 **Population, other specified**

e2159 **Population, unspecified**

e220   Flora and fauna
Plants and animals.

Exclusions: domesticated animals (e350); population (e215)

e2200   **Plants**
Any of various photosynthetic, eukaryotic, multicellular
organisms of the kingdom Plantae characteristically producing
embryos, containing chloroplasts, having cellulose cell walls,
and lacking the power of locomotion, such as trees, flowers,
shrubs and vines.

e2201   **Animals**
Multicellular organisms of the kingdom Animalia, differing
from plants in certain typical characteristics such as capacity
for locomotion, non-photosynthetic metabolism, pronounced
response to stimuli, restricted growth, and fixed bodily
structure, such as wild or farm animals, reptiles, birds, fish and
mammals.

Exclusions: assets (e165); domesticated animals (e350)

e2208   **Fauna and flora, other specified**

e2209   **Fauna and flora, unspecified**

e225   Climate
Meteorological features and events, such as the weather.

*Inclusions: temperature, humidity, atmospheric pressure, precipitation,
wind and seasonal variations*

e2250   **Temperature**
Degree of heat or cold, such as high and low temperature,
normal or extreme temperature.

e2251   **Humidity**
Level of moisture in the air, such as high or low humidity.

e2252   **Atmospheric pressure**
Pressure of the surrounding air, such as pressure related to
height above sea level or meteorological conditions.

e2253   **Precipitation**
Falling of moisture, such as rain, dew, snow, sleet and hail.

e2254 Wind
Air in more or less rapid natural motion, such as a breeze, gale or gust.

e2255 Seasonal variation
Natural, regular and predictable changes from one season to the next, such as summer, autumn, winter and spring.

e2258 Climate, other specified

e2259 Climate, unspecified

e230 Natural events
Geographic and atmospheric changes that cause disruption in an individual's physical environment, occurring regularly or irregularly, such as earthquakes and severe or violent weather conditions, e.g. tornadoes, hurricanes, typhoons, floods, forest fires and ice-storms.

e235 Human-caused events
Alterations or disturbances in the natural environment, caused by humans, that may result in the disruption of people's day-to-day lives, including events or conditions linked to conflict and wars, such as the displacement of people, destruction of social infrastructure, homes and lands, environmental disasters and land, water or air pollution (e.g. toxic spills).

e240 Light
Electromagnetic radiation by which things are made visible by either sunlight or artificial lighting (e.g. candles, oil or paraffin lamps, fires and electricity), and which may provide useful or distracting information about the world.

Inclusions: light intensity; light quality; colour contrasts

e2400 Light intensity
Level or amount of energy being emitted by either a natural (e.g. sun) or an artificial source of light.

e2401 Light quality
The nature of the light being provided and related colour contrasts created in the visual surroundings, and which may provide useful information about the world (e.g. visual information on the presence of stairs or a door) or distractions (e.g. too many visual images).

e2408 Light, other specified

e 2409   Light, unspecified

e 245   Time-related changes
Natural, regular or predictable temporal change.

Inclusions: day/night and lunar cycles

e 2450   Day/night cycles
Natural, regular and predictable changes from day through to
night and back to day, such as day, night, dawn and dusk.

e 2451   Lunar cycles
Natural, regular and predictable changes of the moon's
position in relation to the earth.

e 2458   Time-related changes, other specified

e 2459   Time-related changes, unspecified

e 250   Sound
A phenomenon that is or may be heard, such as banging, ringing,
thumping, singing, whistling, yelling or buzzing, in any volume, timbre
or tone, and that may provide useful or distracting information about
the world.

Inclusions: sound intensity; sound quality

e 2500   Sound intensity
Level or volume of auditory phenomenon determined by the
amount of energy being generated, where high energy levels are
perceived as loud sounds and low energy levels as soft sounds.

e 2501   Sound quality
Nature of a sound as determined by the wavelength and wave
pattern of the sound and perceived as the timbre and tone,
such as harshness or melodiousness, and which may provide
useful information about the world (e.g. sound of dog barking
versus a cat miaowing) or distractions (e.g. background noise).

e 2508   Sound, other specified

e 2509   Sound, unspecified

e 255   Vibration
Regular or irregular to and fro motion of an object or an individual
caused by a physical disturbance, such as shaking, quivering, quick jerky
movements of things, buildings or people caused by small or large
equipment, aircraft and explosions.

*Exclusion: natural events (e230), such as vibration or shaking of the earth
caused by earthquakes*

e 260   Air quality
Characteristics of the atmosphere (outside buildings) or enclosed areas
of air (inside buildings), and which may provide useful or distracting
information about the world.

Inclusions: indoor and outdoor air quality

e 2600   Indoor air quality
Nature of the air inside buildings or enclosed areas, as
determined by odour, smoke, humidity, air conditioning
(controlled air quality) or uncontrolled air quality, and which
may provide useful information about the world (e.g. smell of
leaking gas) or distractions (e.g. overpowering smell of
perfume).

e 2601   Outdoor air quality
Nature of the air outside buildings or enclosed areas, as
determined by odour, smoke, humidity, ozone levels, and
other features of the atmosphere, and which may provide
useful information about the world (e.g. smell of rain) or
distractions (e.g. toxic smells).

e 2608   Air quality, other specified

e 2609   Air quality, unspecified

e 298   Natural environment and human-made changes to environment,
other specified

e 299   Natural environment and human-made changes to environment,
unspecified

Chapter 3
Support and relationships

This chapter is about people or animals that provide practical physical or emotional support, nurturing, protection, assistance and relationships to other persons, in their home, place of work, school or at play or in other aspects of their daily activities. The chapter does not encompass the attitudes of the person or people that are providing the support. The environmental factor being described is not the person or animal, but the amount of physical and emotional support the person or animal provides.

e310 **Immediate family**
Individuals related by birth, marriage or other relationship recognized by the culture as immediate family, such as spouses, partners, parents, siblings, children, foster parents, adoptive parents and grandparents.

Exclusions: extended family (e315); personal care providers and personal assistants (e340)

e315 **Extended family**
Individuals related through family or marriage or other relationships recognized by the culture as extended family, such as aunts, uncles, nephews and nieces.

Exclusion: immediate family (e310)

e320 **Friends**
Individuals who are close and ongoing participants in relationships characterized by trust and mutual support.

e325 **Acquaintances, peers, colleagues, neighbours and community members**
Individuals who are familiar to each other as acquaintances, peers, colleagues, neighbours, and community members, in situations of work, school, recreation, or other aspects of life, and who share demographic features such as age, gender, religious creed or ethnicity or pursue common interests.

Exclusions: associations and organizational services (e5550)

e330 **People in positions of authority**
Individuals who have decision-making responsibilities for others and who have socially defined influence or power based on their social, economic, cultural or religious roles in society, such as teachers, employers, supervisors, religious leaders, substitute decision-makers, guardians or trustees.

e335 **People in subordinate positions**
Individuals whose day-to-day life is influenced by people in positions of authority in work, school or other settings, such as students, workers and members of a religious group.

Exclusion: immediate family (e310)

e340 **Personal care providers and personal assistants**
Individuals who provide services as required to support individuals in their daily activities and maintenance of performance at work, education or other life situation, provided either through public or private funds, or else on a voluntary basis, such as providers of support for home-making and maintenance, personal assistants, transport assistants, paid help, nannies and others who function as primary caregivers.

Exclusions: immediate family (e310); extended family (e315); friends (e320); general social support services (e5750); health professionals (e355)

e345 **Strangers**
Individuals who are unfamiliar and unrelated, or those who have not yet established a relationship or association, including persons unknown to the individual but who are sharing a life situation with them, such as substitute teachers co-workers or care providers.

e350 **Domesticated animals**
Animals that provide physical, emotional, or psychological support, such as pets (dogs, cats, birds, fish, etc.) and animals for personal mobility and transportation.

Exclusions: animals (e2201); assets (e165)

e355 **Health professionals**
All service providers working within the context of the health system, such as doctors, nurses, physiotherapists, occupational therapists, speech therapists, audiologists, orthotist-prosthetists, medical social workers.

Exclusion: other professionals (e360)

e360 **Other professionals**
All service providers working outside the health system, including social workers, lawyers, teachers, architects, and designers.

Exclusion: health professionals (e355)

e398 **Support and relationships, other specified**

e399 Support and relationships, unspecified

Chapter 4

Attitudes

This chapter is about the attitudes that are the observable consequences of customs, practices, ideologies, values, norms, factual beliefs and religious beliefs. These attitudes influence individual behaviour and social life at all levels, from interpersonal relationships and community associations to political, economic and legal structures; for example, individual or societal attitudes about a person's trustworthiness and value as a human being may motivate positive, honorific practices or negative and discriminatory practices (e.g. stigmatizing, stereotyping and marginalizing or neglect of the person).   The attitudes classified are those of people external to the person whose situation is being described. They are not those of the person themselves. The individual attitudes are categorized according to the kinds of relationships listed in Environmental Factors Chapter 3. Values and beliefs are not coded separately from attitudes as they are assumed to be the driving forces behind the attitudes.

e410 **Individual attitudes of immediate family members**
General or specific opinions and beliefs of immediate family members about the person or about other matters (e.g. social, political and economic issues), that influence individual behaviour and actions.

e415 **Individual attitudes of extended family members**
General or specific opinions and beliefs of extended family members about the person or about other matters (e.g. social, political and economic issues), that influence individual behaviour and actions.

e420 **Individual attitudes of friends**
General or specific opinions and beliefs of friends about the person or about other matters (e.g. social, political and economic issues), that influence individual behaviour and actions.

e425 **Individual attitudes of acquaintances, peers, colleagues, neighbours and community members**
General or specific opinions and beliefs of acquaintances, peers, colleagues, neighbours and community members about the person or about other matters (e.g. social, political and economic issues), that influence individual behaviour and actions.

e430 **Individual attitudes of people in positions of authority**
General or specific opinions and beliefs of people in positions of authority about the person or about other matters (e.g. social, political and economic issues), that influence individual behaviour and actions.

e435 **Individual attitudes of people in subordinate positions**
General or specific opinions and beliefs of people in subordinate
positions about the person or about other matters (e.g. social, political
and economic issues), that influence individual behaviour and actions.

e440 **Individual attitudes of personal care providers and personal
assistants**
General or specific opinions and beliefs of personal care providers and
personal assistants about the person or about other matters (e.g. social,
political and economic issues), that influence individual behaviour and
actions.

e445 **Individual attitudes of strangers**
General or specific opinions and beliefs of strangers about the person or
about other matters (e.g. social, political and economic issues), that
influence individual behaviour and actions.

e450 **Individual attitudes of health professionals**
General or specific opinions and beliefs of health professionals about the
person or about other matters (e.g. social, political and economic
issues), that influence individual behaviour and actions.

e455 **Individual attitudes of other professionals**
General or specific opinions and beliefs of health-related and other
professionals about the person or about other matters (e.g. social,
political and economic issues), that influence individual behaviour and
actions.

e460 **Societal attitudes**
General or specific opinions and beliefs generally held by people of a
culture, society, subcultural or other social group about other
individuals or about other social, political and economic issues, that
influence group or individual behaviour and actions.

e465 **Social norms, practices and ideologies**
Customs, practices, rules and abstract systems of values and normative
beliefs (e.g. ideologies, normative world views and moral philosophies)
that arise within social contexts and that affect or create societal and
individual practices and behaviours, such as social norms of moral and
religious behaviour or etiquette; religious doctrine and resulting norms
and practices; norms governing rituals or social gatherings.

e498 **Attitudes, other specified**

e499 **Attitudes, unspecified**

Chapter 5
Services, systems and policies

This chapter is about:

1. *Services* that provide benefits, structured programmes and operations, in various sectors of society, designed to meet the needs of individuals. (Included in services are the people who provide them.) Services may be public, private or voluntary, and may be established at a local, community, regional, state, provincial, national or international level by individuals, associations, organizations, agencies or governments. The goods provided by these services may be general or adapted and specially designed.

2. *Systems* that are administrative control and organizational mechanisms, and are established by governments at the local, regional, national, and international levels, or by other recognized authorities. These systems are designed to organize, control and monitor services that provide benefits, structured programmes and operations in various sectors of society.

3. *Policies* constituted by rules, regulations, conventions and standards established by governments at the local, regional, national, and international levels, or by other recognized authorities. Policies govern and regulate the systems that organize, control and monitor services, structured programmes and operations in various sectors of society.

e510 **Services, systems and policies for the production of consumer goods**
Services, systems and policies that govern and provide for the production of objects and products consumed or used by people.

    e5100 **Services for the production of consumer goods**
Services and programmes for the collection, creation, production and manufacturing of consumer goods and products, such as for products and technology used for mobility, communication, education, transportation, employment and housework, including those who provide these services.

Exclusions: education and training services (e5850); communication services (e5350); Chapter 1

    e5101 **Systems for the production of consumer goods**
Administrative control and monitoring mechanisms, such as regional, national or international organizations that set standards (e.g. International Organization for Standardization) and consumer bodies, that govern the collection, creation, production and manufacturing of consumer goods and products.

e5102   **Policies for the production of consumer goods**
Legislation, regulations and standards for the collection,
creation, production and manufacturing of consumer goods
and products, such as which standards to adopt.

e5108   **Services, systems and policies for the production of
consumer goods, other specified**

e5109   **Services, systems and policies for the production of
consumer goods, unspecified**

e515 **Architecture and construction services, systems and policies**
Services, systems and policies for the design and construction of
buildings, public and private.

Exclusion: open space planning services, systems and policies (e520)

e5150   **Architecture and construction services**
Services and programmes for design, construction and
maintenance of residential, commercial, industrial and public
buildings, such as house-building, the operationalization of
design principles, building codes, regulations and standards,
including those who provide these services.

e5151   **Architecture and construction systems**
Administrative control and monitoring mechanisms that
govern the planning, design, construction and maintenance of
residential, commercial, industrial and public buildings, such
as for implementing and monitoring building codes,
construction standards, and fire and life safety standards.

e5152   **Architecture and construction policies**
Legislation, regulations and standards that govern the
planning, design, construction and maintenance of residential,
commercial, industrial and public buildings, such as policies
on building codes, construction standards, and fire and life
safety standards.

e5158   **Architecture and construction services, systems and
policies, other specified**

e5159   **Architecture and construction services, systems and
policies, unspecified**

e520 Open space planning services, systems and policies
Services, systems and policies for the planning, design, development and maintenance of public lands, (e.g. parks, forests, shorelines, wetlands) and private lands in the rural, suburban and urban context.

Exclusion: architecture and construction services, systems and policies (e515)

e5200 **Open space planning services**
Services and programmes aimed at planning, creating and maintaining urban, suburban, rural, recreational, conservation and environmental space, meeting and commercial open spaces (plazas, open-air markets) and pedestrian and vehicular transportation routes for intended uses, including those who provide these services.

Exclusions: products for design, building and construction for public (e150) and private (e155) use; products of land development (e160)

e5201 **Open space planning systems**
Administrative control and monitoring mechanisms, such as for the implementation of local, regional or national planning acts, design codes, heritage or conservation policies and environmental planning policy, that govern the planning, design, development and maintenance of open space, including rural, suburban and urban land, parks, conservation areas and wildlife reserves.

e5202 **Open space planning policies**
Legislation, regulations and standards that govern the planning, design, development and maintenance of open space, including rural land, suburban land, urban land, parks, conservation areas and wildlife reserves, such as local, regional or national planning acts, design codes, heritage or conservation policies, and environmental planning policies.

e5208 **Open space planning services, systems and policies, other specified**

e5209 **Open space planning services, systems and policies, unspecified**

e525 Housing services, systems and policies
Services, systems and policies for the provision of shelters, dwellings or lodging for people.

e5250   Housing services
Services and programmes aimed at locating, providing and
maintaining houses or shelters for persons to live in, such as
estate agencies, housing organizations, shelters for homeless
people, including those who provide these services.

e5251   Housing systems
Administrative control and monitoring mechanisms that
govern housing or sheltering of people, such as systems for
implementing and monitoring housing policies.

e5252   Housing policies
Legislation, regulations and standards that govern housing or
sheltering of people, such as legislation and policies for
determination of eligibility for housing or shelter, policies
concerning government involvement in developing and
maintaining housing, and policies concerning how and where
housing is developed.

e5258   Housing services, systems and policies, other specified

e5259   Housing services, systems and policies, unspecified

e530   Utilities services, systems and policies
Services, systems and policies for publicly provided utilities, such as
water, fuel, electricity, sanitation, public transportation and essential
services.

Exclusion: civil protection services, systems and policies (e545)

e5300   Utilities services
Services and programmes supplying the population as a whole
with essential energy (e.g. fuel and electricity), sanitation, water
and other essential services (e.g. emergency repair services) for
residential and commercial consumers, including those who
provide these services.

e5301   Utilities systems
Administrative control and monitoring mechanisms that
govern the provision of utilities services, such as health and
safety boards and consumer councils.

e 5302   Utilities policies
Legislation, regulations and standards that govern the
provision of utilities services, such as health and safety
standards governing delivery and supply of water and fuel,
sanitation practices in communities, and policies for other
essential services and supply during shortages or natural
disasters.

e 5308   Utilities services, systems and policies, other specified

e 5309   Utilities services, systems and policies, unspecified

e535   Communication services, systems and policies
Services, systems and policies for the transmission and exchange of
information.

e 5350   Communication services
Services and programmes aimed at transmitting information
by a variety of methods such as telephone, fax, surface and air
mail, electronic mail and other computer-based systems (e.g.
telephone relay, teletype, teletext, and internet services),
including those who provide these services.

Exclusion: media services (e5600)

e 5351   Communication systems
Administrative control and monitoring mechanisms, such as
telecommunication regulation authorities and other such
bodies, that govern the transmission of information by a
variety of methods, including telephone, fax, surface and air
mail, electronic mail and computer-based systems.

e 5352   Communication policies
Legislation, regulations and standards that govern the
transmission of information by a variety of methods including
telephone, fax, post office, electronic mail and computer-based
systems, such as eligibility for access to communication
services, requirements for a postal address, and standards for
provision of telecommunications.

**e 5358   Communication services, systems and policies, other
specified**

e 5359   Communication services, systems and policies, unspecified

e540   Transportation services, systems and policies
Services, systems and policies for enabling people or goods to move or
be moved from one location to another.

e5400   Transportation services
Services and programmes aimed at moving persons or goods by road, paths, rail, air or water, by public or private transport, including those who provide these services.

Exclusion: products for personal mobility and transportation (e115)

e5401   Transportation systems
Administrative control and monitoring mechanisms that govern the moving of persons or goods by road, paths, rail, air or water, such as systems for determining eligibility for operating vehicles and, implementation and monitoring of health and safety standards related to use of different types of transportation.

Exclusion: social security services, systems and policies (e570)

e5402   Transportation policies
Legislation, regulations and standards that govern the moving of persons or goods by road, paths, rail, air or water, such as transportation planning acts and policies, policies for the provision and access to public transportation.

e5408   Transportation services, systems and policies, other specified

e5409   Transportation services, systems and policies, unspecified

e545   Civil protection services, systems and policies
Services, systems and policies aimed at safeguarding people and property.

Exclusion: utilities services, systems and policies (e530)

e5450   Civil protection services
Services and programmes organized by the community and aimed at safeguarding people and property, such as fire, police, emergency and ambulance services, including those who provide these services.

e5451   Civil protection systems
Administrative control and monitoring mechanisms that govern the safeguarding of people and property, such as systems by which provision of police, fire, emergency and ambulance services are organized.

e5452   **Civil protection policies**
Legislation, regulations and standards that govern the
safeguarding of people and property, such as policies
governing provision of police, fire, emergency and ambulance
services.

e5458   **Civil protection services, systems and policies, other
specified**

e5459   **Civil protection services, systems and policies, unspecified**

e550   **Legal services, systems and policies**
Services, systems and policies concerning the legislation and other law
of a country.

e5500   **Legal services**
Services and programmes aimed at providing the authority of
the state as defined in law, such as courts, tribunals and other
agencies for hearing and settling civil litigation and criminal
trials, attorney representation, services of notaries, mediation,
arbitration and correctional or penal facilities, including those
who provide these services.

e5501   **Legal systems**
Administrative control and monitoring mechanisms that
govern the administration of justice, such as systems for
implementing and monitoring formal rules (e.g. laws,
regulations, customary law, religious law, international laws
and conventions).

e5502   **Legal policies**
Legislation, regulations and standards, such as laws, customary
law, religious law, international laws and conventions, that
govern the administration of justice.

e5508   **Legal services, systems and policies, other specified**

e5509   **Legal services, systems and policies, unspecified**

e555   **Associations and organizational services, systems and policies**
Services, systems and policies relating to groups of people who have
joined together in the pursuit of common, noncommercial interests,
often with an associated membership structure.

e5550   Associations and organizational services
Services and programmes provided by people who have joined together in the pursuit of common, noncommercial interests with people who have the same interests, where the provision of such services may be tied to membership, such as associations and organizations providing recreation and leisure, sporting, cultural, religious and mutual aid services.

e5551   Associations and organizational systems
Administrative control and monitoring mechanisms that govern the relationships and activities of people coming together with common noncommercial interests and the establishment and conduct of associations and organizations such as mutual aid organizations, recreational and leisure organizations, cultural and religious associations and not-for-profit organizations.

e5552   Associations and organizational policies
Legislation, regulations and standards that govern the relationships and activities of people coming together with common noncommercial interests, such as policies that govern the establishment and conduct of associations and organizations, including mutual aid organizations, recreational and leisure organizations, cultural and religious associations and not-for-profit organizations.

e5558   Associations and organizational services, systems and policies, other specified

e5559   Associations and organizational services, systems and policies, unspecified

e560   Media services, systems and policies
Services, systems and policies for the provision of mass communication through radio, television, newspapers and internet.

e5600   Media services
Services and programmes aimed at providing mass communication, such as radio, television, closed captioning services, press reporting services, newspapers, Braille services and computer-based mass communication (world wide web, internet), including those who provide these services.

Exclusion: communication services (e5350)

e 5601   Media systems
Administrative control and monitoring mechanisms that
govern the provision of news and information to the general
public, such as standards that govern the content, distribution,
dissemination, access to and methods of communicating via
radio, television, press reporting services, newspapers and
computer-based mass communication (world wide web,
internet).

*Inclusions: requirements to provide closed captions on
television, Braille versions of newspapers or other publications,
and teletext radio transmissions*

Exclusion: communication systems (e5351)

e 5602   Media policies
Legislation, regulations and standards that govern the
provision of news and information to the general public, such
as policies that govern the content, distribution, dissemination,
access to and methods of communicating via radio, television,
press reporting services, newspapers and computer-based mass
communication (world wide web, internet).

Exclusion: communication policies (e5352)

e 5608   Media services, systems and policies, other specified

e 5609   Media services, systems and policies, unspecified

e 565   **Economic services, systems and policies**
Services, systems and policies related to the overall system of
production, distribution, consumption and use of goods and services.

Exclusion: social security services, systems and policies (e570)

e 5650   Economic services
Services and programmes aimed at the overall production,
distribution, consumption and use of goods and services, such
as the private commercial sector (e.g. businesses, corporations,
private for-profit ventures), the public sector (e.g. public,
commercial services such as cooperatives and corporations),
financial organizations (e.g. banks and insurance services),
including those who provide these services.

*Exclusions: utilities services (e5300); labour and employment
services (e5900)*

e5651   Economic systems
Administrative control and monitoring mechanisms that
govern the production, distribution, consumption and use of
goods and services, such as systems for implementing and
monitoring economic policies.

*Exclusions: utilities systems (e5301); labour and employment
systems (e5901)*

e5652   Economic policies
Legislation, regulations and standards that govern the
production, distribution, consumption and use of goods and
services, such as economic doctrines adopted and
implemented by governments.

*Exclusions: utilities policies (e5302); labour and employment
policies (e5902)*

e5658   Economic services, systems and policies, other specified

e5659   Economic services, systems and policies, unspecified

e570   **Social security services, systems and policies**
Services, systems and policies aimed at providing income support to
people who, because of age, poverty, unemployment, health condition
or disability, require public assistance that is funded either by general
tax revenues or contributory schemes.

Exclusion: economic services, systems and policies (e565)

e5700   Social security services
Services and programmes aimed at providing income support
to people who, because of age, poverty, unemployment, health
condition or disability, require public assistance that is funded
either by general tax revenues or contributory schemes, such as
services for determining eligibility, delivering or distributing
assistance payments for the following types of programmes:
social assistance programmes (e.g. non-contributory welfare,
poverty or other needs-based compensation), social insurance
programmes (e.g. contributory accident or unemployment
insurance), and disability and related pension schemes (e.g.
income replacement), including those who provide these
services.

Exclusions: health services (e5800)

e 5701   **Social security systems**
Administrative control and monitoring mechanisms that
govern the programmes and schemes that provide income
support to people who, because of age, poverty,
unemployment, health condition or disability, require public
assistance, such as systems for the implementation of rules and
regulations governing the eligibility for social assistance,
welfare, unemployment insurance payments, pensions and
disability benefits.

e 5702   **Social security policies**
Legislation, regulations and standards that govern the
programmes and schemes that provide income support to
people who, because of age, poverty, unemployment, health
condition or disability, require public assistance, such as
legislation and regulations governing the eligibility for social
assistance, welfare, unemployment insurance payments,
disability and related pensions and disability benefits.

e 5708   **Social security services, systems and policies, other specified**

e 5709   **Social security services, systems and policies, unspecified**

e 575   **General social support services, systems and policies**
Services, systems and policies aimed at providing support to those
requiring assistance in areas such as shopping, housework, transport,
self-care and care of others, in order to function more fully in society.

*Exclusions: social security services, systems and policies (e570); personal
care providers and personal assistants (e340); health services, systems and
policies (e580)*

e 5750   **General social support services**
Services and programmes aimed at providing social support to
people who, because of age, poverty, unemployment, health
condition or disability, require public assistance in the areas of
shopping, housework, transport, self-care and care of others, in
order to function more fully in society.

e 5751   **General social support systems**
Administrative control and monitoring mechanisms that
govern the programmes and schemes that provide social
support to people who, because of age, poverty,
unemployment, health condition or disability, require such
support, including systems for the implementation of rules and
regulations governing eligibility for social support services and
the provision of these services.

e5752   General social support policies
Legislation, regulations and standards that govern the
programme and schemes that provide social support to people
who, because of age, poverty, unemployment, health condition
or disability, require such support, including legislation and
regulations governing eligibility for social support.

**e5758   General social support services, systems and policies, other
specified**

**e5759   General social support services, systems and policies,
unspecified**

e580   Health services, systems and policies
Services, systems and policies for preventing and treating health
problems, providing medical rehabilitation and promoting a healthy
lifestyle.

Exclusion: general social support services, systems and policies (e575)

e5800   Health services
Services and programmes at a local, community, regional, state
or national level, aimed at delivering interventions to
individuals for their physical, psychological and social well-
being, such as health promotion and disease prevention
services, primary care services, acute care, rehabilitation and
long-term care services; services that are publicly or privately
funded, delivered on a short-term, long-term, periodic or one-
time basis, in a variety of service settings such as community,
home-based, school and work settings, general hospitals,
speciality hospitals, clinics, and residential and non-residential
care facilities, including those who provide these services.

e5801   Health systems
Administrative control and monitoring mechanisms that
govern the range of services provided to individuals for their
physical, psychological and social well-being, in a variety of
settings including community, home-based, school and work
settings, general hospitals, speciality hospitals, clinics, and
residential and non-residential care facilities, such as systems
for implementing regulations and standards that determine
eligibility for services, provision of devices, assistive technology
or other adapted equipment, and legislation such as health acts
that govern features of a health system such as accessibility,
universality, portability, public funding and
comprehensiveness.

e5802   **Health policies**
Legislation, regulations and standards that govern the range of
services provided to individuals for their physical,
psychological and social well-being, in a variety of settings
including community, home-based, school and work settings,
general hospitals, speciality hospitals, clinics, and residential
and non-residential care facilities, such as policies and
standards that determine eligibility for services, provision of
devices, assistive technology or other adapted equipment, and
legislation such as health acts that govern features of a health
system such as accessibility, universality, portability, public
funding and comprehensiveness.

e5808   **Health services, systems and policies, other specified**

e5809   **Health services, systems and policies, unspecified**

e585   **Education and training services, systems and policies**
Services, systems and policies for the acquisition, maintenance and
improvement of knowledge, expertise and vocational or artistic skills.
See UNESCO's International Standard Classification of Education
(ISCED-1997).

e5850   **Education and training services**
Services and programmes concerned with education and the
acquisition, maintenance and improvement of knowledge,
expertise and vocational or artistic skills, such as those
provided for different levels of education (e.g. preschool,
primary school, secondary school, post-secondary institutions,
professional programmes, training and skills programmes,
apprenticeships and continuing education), including those
who provide these services.

e5851   **Education and training systems**
Administrative control and monitoring mechanisms that
govern the delivery of education programmes, such as systems
for the implementation of policies and standards that
determine eligibility for public or private education and special
needs-based programmes; local, regional or national boards of
education or other authoritative bodies that govern features of
the education systems, including curricula, size of classes,
numbers of schools in a region, fees and subsidies, special meal
programmes and after-school care services.

e 5852   **Education and training policies**
Legislation, regulations and standards that govern the delivery of education programme, such as policies and standards that determine eligibility for public or private education and special needs-based programmes, and dictate the structure of local, regional or national boards of education or other authoritative bodies that govern features of the education system, including curricula, size of classes, numbers of schools in a region, fees and subsidies, special meal programmes and after-school care services.

e 5858   **Education and training services, systems and policies, other specified**

e 5859   **Education and training services, systems and policies, unspecified**

e 590   **Labour and employment services, systems and policies**
Services, systems and policies related to finding suitable work for persons who are unemployed or looking for different work, or to support individuals already employed who are seeking promotion.

Exclusion: economic services, systems and policies (e565)

e 5900   **Labour and employment services**
Services and programmes provided by local, regional or national governments, or private organizations to find suitable work for persons who are unemployed or looking for different work, or to support individuals already employed, such as services of employment search and preparation, reemployment, job placement, outplacement, vocational follow-up, occupational health and safety services, and work environment services (e.g. ergonomics, human resources and personnel management services, labour relations services, professional association services), including those who provide these services.

e 5901   **Labour and employment systems**
Administrative control and monitoring mechanisms that govern the distribution of occupations and other forms of remunerative work in the economy, such as systems for implementing policies and standards for employment creation, employment security, designated and competitive employment, labour standards and law, and trade unions.

    e5902   **Labour and employment policies**
Legislation, regulations and standards that govern the
distribution of occupations and other forms of remunerative
work in the economy, such as standards and policies for
employment creation, employment security, designated and
competitive employment, labour standards and law, and trade
unions.

    e5908   **Labour and employment services, systems and policies,
other specified**

    e5909   **Labour and employment services, systems and policies,
unspecified**

e595   **Political services, systems and policies**
Services, systems and policies related to voting, elections and
governance of countries, regions and communities, as well as
international organizations.

    e5950   **Political services**
Services and structures such as local, regional and national
governments, international organizations and the people who
are elected or nominated to positions within these structures,
such as the United Nations, European Union, governments,
regional authorities, local village authorities, traditional
leaders.

    e5951   **Political systems**
Structures and related operations that organise political and
economic power in a society, such as executive and legislative
branches of government, and the constitutional or other legal
sources from which they derive their authority, such as political
organizational doctrine, constitutions, agencies of executive
and legislative branches of government, the military.

    e5952   **Political policy**
Laws and policies formulated and enforced through political
systems that govern the operation of the political system, such
as policies governing election campaigns, registration of
political parties, voting, and members in international political
organizations, including treaties, constitutional and other law
governing legislation and regulation.

    e5958   **Political services, systems and policies, other specified**

    e5959   **Political services, systems and policies, unspecified**

e598   Services, systems and policies, other specified

e 599   Services, systems and policies, unspecified

ICF

Annexes

Annex 1

Taxonomic and terminological issues

The ICF classification is organized in a hierarchical scheme keeping in mind the following standard taxonomic principles:

- The components of Body Functions and Structures, Activities and Participation, and Environmental Factors are classified independently. Hence, a term included under one component is not repeated under another.

- Within each component, the categories are arranged in a stem–branch–leaf scheme, so that a lower-level category shares the attributes of the higher-level categories of which it is a member.

- Categories are mutually exclusive, i.e. no two categories at the same level share exactly the same attributes. However, this should not be confused with the use of more than one category to classify a particular individual's functioning. Such a practice is allowed, indeed encouraged, where necessary.

1. Terms for categories in ICF

Terms are the designation of defined concepts in linguistic expressions, such as words or phrases. Most of the terms over which confusion arises are used with common-sense meanings in everyday speech and writing. For example, impairment, disability and handicap are often used interchangeably in everyday contexts, although in the 1980 version of ICIDH these terms had stipulated definitions, which gave them a precisely defined meaning. During the revision process, the term "handicap" was abandoned and "disability" was used as an umbrella term for all three perspectives - body, individual and societal. Clarity and precision, however, are needed to define the various concepts, so that appropriate terms may be chosen to express each of the underlying concepts unambiguously. This is particularly important because ICF, as a written classification, will be translated into many languages. Beyond a common understanding of the concepts, it is also essential that an agreement be reached on the term that best reflects the content in each language. There may be many alternatives, and decisions should be made based on accuracy, acceptability, and overall usefulness. It is hoped that the usefulness of ICF will go in parallel with its clarity.

With this aim in mind, notes on some of the terms used in ICF follow:

Well-being is a general term encompassing the total universe of human life domains, including physical, mental and social aspects, that make up what can be called a "good life". Health domains are a subset of domains that make up the total universe of human life. This relationship is presented in the following diagram representing well-being:

Fig. 1   The universe of well-being

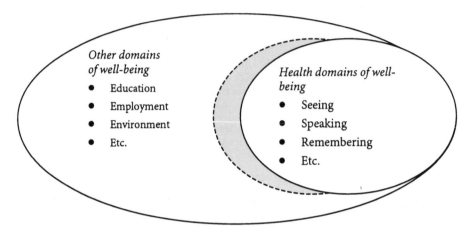

Health states and health domains: A health state is the level of functioning within a given health domain of ICF. Health domains denote areas of life that are interpreted to be within the "health" notion, such as those which, for health systems purposes, can be defined as the primary responsibility of the health system. ICF does not dictate a fixed boundary between health and health-related domains. There may be a grey zone depending on differing conceptualizations of health and health-related elements which can then be mapped onto the ICF domains.

Health-related states and health-related domains: A health-related state is the level of functioning within a given health-related domain of ICF. Health-related domains are those areas of functioning that, while they have a strong relationship to a health condition, are not likely to be the primary responsibility of the health system, but rather of other systems contributing to overall well-being. In ICF, only those domains of well-being related to health are covered.

Health condition is an umbrella term for disease (acute or chronic), disorder, injury or trauma. A health condition may also include other circumstances such as pregnancy, ageing, stress, congenital anomaly, or genetic predisposition. Health conditions are coded using ICD-10.

Functioning is an umbrella term for body functions, body structures, activities and participation. It denotes the positive aspects of the interaction between an individual (with a health condition) and that individual's contextual factors (environmental and personal factors).

Disability is an umbrella term for impairments, activity limitations and participation restrictions. It denotes the negative aspects of the interaction between an individual (with a health condition) and that individual's contextual factors (environmental and personal factors).

Body functions are the physiological functions of body systems, including psychological functions. "Body" refers to the human organism as a whole, and thus includes the brain. Hence, mental (or psychological) functions are subsumed under body functions. The standard for these functions is considered to be the statistical norm for humans.

Body structures are the structural or anatomical parts of the body such as organs, limbs and their components classified according to body systems. The standard for these structures is considered to be the statistical norm for humans.

Impairment is a loss or abnormality in body structure or physiological function (including mental functions). Abnormality here is used strictly to refer to a significant variation from established statistical norms (i.e. as a deviation from a population mean within measured standard norms) and should be used only in this sense.

Activity is the execution of a task or action by an individual. It represents the individual perspective of functioning.

Activity limitations[18] are difficulties an individual may have in executing activities. An activity limitation may range from a slight to a severe deviation in terms of quality or quantity in executing the activity in a manner or to the extent that is expected of people without the health condition.

Participation is a person's involvement in a life situation. It represents the societal perspective of functioning.

Participation restrictions[19] are problems an individual may experience in involvement in life situations. The presence of a participation restriction is determined by comparing an individual's participation to that which is expected of an individual without disability in that culture or society.

Contextual factors are the factors that together constitute the complete context of an individual's life, and in particular the background against which health states are classified in ICF. There are two components of contextual factors: Environmental Factors and Personal Factors.

Environmental factors constitute a component of ICF, and refer to all aspects of the external or extrinsic world that form the context of an individual's life and, as such, have an impact on that person's functioning. Environmental factors include

---

[18] "Activity limitation" replaces the term "disability" used in the 1980 version of ICIDH.

[19] "Participation restriction" replaces the term "handicap" used in the 1980 version of ICIDH.

the physical world and its features, the human-made physical world, other people in different relationships and roles, attitudes and values, social systems and services, and policies, rules and laws.

Personal factors are contextual factors that relate to the individual such as age, gender, social status, life experiences and so on, which are not currently classified in ICF but which users may incorporate in their applications of the classification.

Facilitators are factors in a person's environment that, through their absence or presence, improve functioning and reduce disability. These include aspects such as a physical environment that is accessible, the availability of relevant assistive technology, and positive attitudes of people towards disability, as well as services, systems and policies that aim to increase the involvement of all people with a health condition in all areas of life. Absence of a factor can also be facilitating, for example the absence of stigma or negative attitudes. Facilitators can prevent an impairment or activity limitation from becoming a participation restriction, since the actual performance of an action is enhanced, despite the person's problem with capacity.

Barriers are factors in a person's environment that, through their absence or presence, limit functioning and create disability. These include aspects such as a physical environment that is inaccessible, lack of relevant assistive technology, and negative attitudes of people towards disability, as well as services, systems and policies that are either nonexistent or that hinder the involvement of all people with a health condition in all areas of life.

Capacity is a construct that indicates, as a qualifier, the highest probable level of functioning that a person may reach in a domain in the Activities and Participation list at a given moment. Capacity is measured in a uniform or standard environment, and thus reflects the environmentally adjusted ability of the individual. The Environmental Factors component can be used to describe the features of this uniform or standard environment.

Performance is a construct that describes, as a qualifier, what individuals do in their current environment, and so brings in the aspect of a person's involvement in life situations. The current environment is also described using the Environmental Factors component.

Fig. 2   Structure of ICF

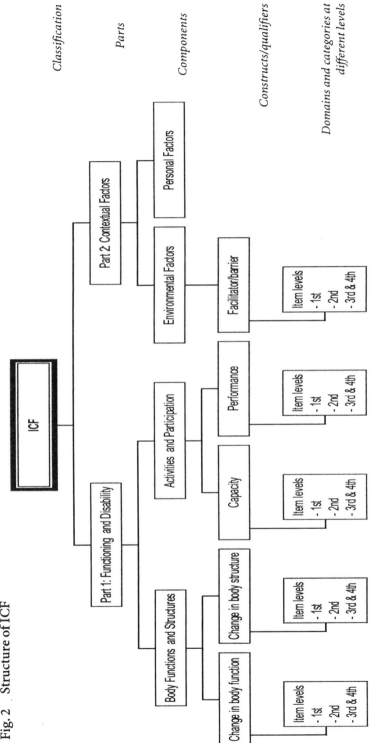

2. ICF as a classification

In order to understand the overall classification of ICF, it is important to understand its structure. This is reflected in the definitions of the following terms and illustrated in Fig. 2.

Classification is the overall structure and universe of ICF. In the hierarchy, this is the top term.

Parts of the classification are each of the two main subdivisions of the classification.

- Part 1 covers Functioning and Disability
- Part 2 covers Contextual Factors.

Components are each of the two main subdivisions of the parts.

The components of Part 1 are:

- Body Functions and Structures
- Activities and Participation.

The components of Part 2 are:

- Environmental Factors
- Personal Factors (not classified in ICF).

Constructs are defined through the use of qualifiers with relevant codes.

There are four constructs for Part 1 and one for Part 2.

For Part 1, the constructs are:

- Change in body function
- Change in body structure
- Capacity
- Performance

For Part 2, the construct is:

- Facilitators or barriers in environmental factors

Domains are a practical, meaningful set of related physiological functions, anatomical structures, actions, tasks, or areas of life. Domains make up the different chapters and blocks within each component.

Categories are classes and subclasses within a domain of a component, i.e. units of classification.

Levels make up the hierarchical order providing indications as to the detail of categories (i.e. granularity of the domains and categories). The first level comprises all the second-level items, and so on.

3. Definitions for ICF categories

Definitions are statements that set out the essential attributes (i.e. qualities, properties or relationships) of the concept designated by the category. A definition states what sort of thing or phenomenon the term denotes, and operationally, notes how it differs from other related things or phenomena.

During the construction of the definitions of the ICF categories, the following ideal characteristics of operational definitions, including inclusions and exclusions, were kept in mind:

- Definitions should be meaningful and logically consistent.

- They must uniquely identify the concept intended by the category.

- They must present essential attributes of the concept – both intentional (what the concept signifies intrinsically) and extensional (what objects or phenomena it refers to).

- They should be precise, unambiguous, and cover the full meaning of the term.

- They should be expressed in operational terms (e.g. in terms of severity, duration, relative importance, and possible associations).

- They should avoid circularity, i.e. the term itself, or any synonym for it, should not appear in the definition, nor should it include a term defined elsewhere using the first term in its definition.

- Where appropriate, they should refer to possible etiological or interactive factors.

- They must fit the attributes of the higher-ranking terms (e.g. a third-level term should include the general characteristics of the second-level category to which it belongs).

- They must be consistent with the attributes of the subordinate terms (e.g. the attributes of a second-level term cannot contradict those of third-level terms under it).

- They must not be figurative or metaphorical, but operational.

- They should make empirical statements that are observable, testable or inferable by indirect means.

- They should be expressed in neutral terms as far as possible, without undue negative connotation.

- They should be short and avoid technical terms where possible (with the exception of some Body Functions and Structures terms).

- They should have inclusions that provide synonyms and examples that take into account cultural variation and differences across the life span.

- They should have exclusions to alert users to possible confusion with related terms.

4. Additional note on terminology

Underlying the terminology of any classification is the fundamental distinction between the phenomena being classified and the structure of the classification itself. As a general matter, it is important to distinguish between the world and the terms we use to describe the world. For example, the terms 'dimension' or 'domain' could be precisely defined to refer to the world and 'component' and 'category' defined to refer only to the classification.

At the same time, there is a correspondence (i.e. a matching function) between these terms and it is possible that a wide variety of users may use these terms interchangeably. For more highly specialized requirements, for database construction and research modelling for example, it is essential for users to identify separately, and with a clearly distinct terminology, the elements of the conceptual model and those of the classification structure. Yet, it has been felt that the precision and purity that such an approach provides is not worth the price paid in a level of abstraction that might undermine the usefulness of the ICF, or more importantly to restrict the range of potential users of this classification.

Annex 2

Coding guidelines for ICF

ICF is intended for the coding of different health and health-related states.[20] Users are strongly recommended to read through the Introduction to ICF before studying the coding rules and guidelines. Furthermore, it is highly recommended that users obtain training in the use of the classification through WHO and its network of collaborating centres.

The following are features of the classification that have a bearing on its use.

1. Organization and structure

Parts of the Classification

ICF is organized into two parts.

Part 1 is composed of the following components:

- Body Functions and Body Structures
- Activities and Participation.

Part 2 is composed of the following components:

- Environmental Factors
- Personal Factors (currently not classified in the ICF).

These components are denoted by prefixes in each code.

- *b* for Body Functions and
- *s* for Body Structures
- *d* for Activities and Participation
- *e* for Environmental Factors

The prefix *d* denotes the domains within the component of Activities and Participation. At the user's discretion, the prefix *d* can be replaced by *a* or *p*, to denote activities and participation respectively.

---

[20] The disease itself should not be coded. This can be done using the International Statistical Classification of Diseases and Related Health Problems, Tenth Revision (ICD-10), which is a classification designed to permit the systematic recording, analysis, interpretation and comparison of mortality and morbidity data on diagnoses of diseases and other health problems. Users of ICF are encouraged to use this classification in conjunction with ICD-10 (see page 3 of Introduction regarding overlap between the classifications)

The letters *b, s, d* and *e* are followed by a numeric code that starts with the chapter number (one digit), followed by the second level (two digits), and the third and fourth level[21] (one digit each). For example, in the Body Functions classification there are these codes:

b2	Sensory functions and pain	(first-level item)
b210	Seeing functions	(second-level item)
b2102	Quality of vision	(third-level item)
b21022	Contrast sensitivity	(fourth-level item)

Depending on the user's needs, any number of applicable codes can be employed at each level. To describe an individual's situation, more than one code at each level may be applicable. These may be independent or interrelated.

In ICF, a person's health state may be assigned an array of codes across the domains of the components of the classification. The maximum number of codes available for each application is 34 at the chapter level (8 body functions, 8 body structures, 9 performance and 9 capacity codes), and 362 at the second level. At the third and fourth levels, there are up to 1424 codes available, which together constitute the full version of the classification. In real-life applications of ICF, a set of 3 to 18 codes may be adequate to describe a case with two-level (three-digit) precision. Generally, the more detailed four-level version is intended for specialist services (e.g. rehabilitation outcomes, geriatrics, or mental health), whereas the two-level classification can be used for surveys and health outcome evaluation.

The domains should be coded as applicable to a given moment (i.e. as a snapshot description of an encounter), which is the default position. Use over time, however, is also possible in order to describe a trajectory over time or a process. Users should then identify their coding style and the time-frame that they use.

Chapters

Each component of the classification is organized into chapter and domain headings under which are common categories or specific items. For example, in the Body Functions classification, Chapter 1 deals with all mental functions.

Blocks

The chapters are often subdivided into "blocks" of categories. For example, in Chapter 3 of the Activities and Participation classification (Communication), there are three blocks: Communicating·Receiving (d310–d329), Communicating·Producing (d330–d349), and Conversation and using communication devices and techniques (d350–d369). Blocks are provided as a convenience to the user and, strictly speaking, are not part of the structure of the classification and normally will not be used for coding purposes.

---

[21] Only the Body Functions and Body Structure classifications contain fourth-level items.

Categories

Within each chapter there are individual two-, three- or four-level categories, each with a short definition and inclusions and exclusions as appropriate to assist in the selection of the appropriate code.

Definitions

ICF gives operational definitions of the health and health-related categories, as opposed to "vernacular" or layperson's definitions. These definitions describe the essential attributes of each domain (e.g. qualities, properties, and relationships) and contain information as to what is included and excluded in each category. The definitions also contain commonly used anchor points for assessment, for application in surveys and questionnaires, or alternatively, for the results of assessment instruments coded in ICF terms. For example, visual acuity functions are defined in terms of monocular and binocular acuity at near and far distances so that the severity of visual acuity difficulty can be coded as none, mild, moderate, severe or total.

Inclusion terms

Inclusion terms are listed after the definition of many categories. They are provided as a guide to the content of the category, and are not meant to be exhaustive. In the case of second-level items, the inclusions cover all embedded, third-level items.

Exclusion terms

Exclusion terms are provided where, owing to the similarity with another term, application might prove difficult. For example, it might be thought that the category "Toileting" includes the category "Caring for body parts". To distinguish the two, however, "Toileting" is excluded from category d520 "Caring for body parts" and coded to d530.

Other specified

At the end of each embedded set of third- or fourth-level items, and at the end of each chapter, are "other specified" categories (uniquely identified by the final code number 8). These allow for the coding of aspects of functioning that are not included within any of the other specific categories. When "other specified" is employed, the user should specify the new item in an additional list.

Unspecified

The last categories within each embedded set of third- or fourth-level items, and at the end of each chapter, are "unspecified" categories that allow for the coding of functions that fit within the group but for which there is insufficient information to permit the assignment of a more specific category. This code has the same meaning as the second- or third-level term immediately above, without any additional information (for blocks, the "other specified" and "unspecified" categories are joined into a single item, but are always identified by the final code number 9).

Qualifiers

The ICF codes require the use of one or more qualifiers, which denote, for example, the magnitude of the level of health or severity of the problem at issue. Qualifiers are coded as one, two or more numbers after a point. Use of any code should be accompanied by at least one qualifier. Without qualifiers codes have no inherent meaning (by default, WHO interprets incomplete codes as signifying the absence of a problem -- xxx.00).

The first qualifier for Body Functions and Structures, the performance and capacity qualifiers for Activities and Participation, and the first qualifier for Environmental Factors all describe the extent of problems in the respective component.

All components are quantified using the same generic scale. Having a problem may mean an impairment, limitation, restriction or barrier, depending on the construct. Appropriate qualifying words as shown in brackets below should be chosen according to the relevant classification domain (where xxx stands for the second-level domain number):

xxx.0	NO problem	(none, absent, negligible,…)	0–4 %
xxx.1	MILD problem	(slight, low,…)	5–24 %
xxx.2	MODERATE problem	(medium, fair,...)	25–49 %
xxx.3	SEVERE problem	(high, extreme, …)	50–95 %
xxx.4	COMPLETE problem	(total,…)	96–100 %
xxx.8	not specified		
xxx.9	not applicable		

Broad ranges of percentages are provided for those cases in which calibrated assessment instruments or other standards are available to quantify the impairment, capacity limitation, performance problem or environmental barrier/facilitator. For example, when "no problem" or "complete problem" is coded, this may have a margin of error of up to 5%. A "moderate problem" is defined as up to half of the scale of total difficulty. The percentages are to be calibrated in different domains with reference to population standards as percentiles. For this quantification to be used in a universal manner, assessment procedures have to be developed through research.

In the case of the Environmental Factors component, this first qualifier can also be used to denote the extent of positive aspects of the environment, or facilitators. To denote facilitators, the same 0–4 scale can be used, but the point is replaced by a plus sign: e.g. e110+2. Environmental factors can be coded either (i) in relation to each component; or (ii) without relation to each component (see section 3 below). The first style is preferable since it identifies the impact and attribution more clearly.

Additional qualifiers

For different users, it might be appropriate and helpful to add other kinds of information to the coding of each item. There are a variety of additional qualifiers that could be useful, as mentioned later.

Coding positive aspects

At the user's discretion coding scales can be developed to capture the positive aspects of functioning:

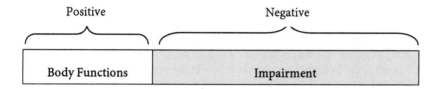

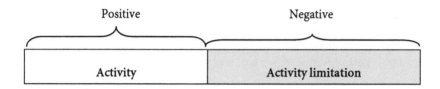

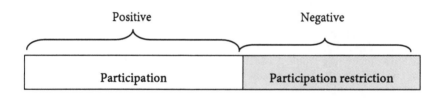

2. General coding rules

The following rules are essential for accurate retrieval of information for the various uses of the classification.

Select an array of codes to form an individual's profile

ICF classifies health and health-related states and therefore requires the assigning of a series of codes that best describe the profile of the person's functioning. ICF is not an "event classification" like ICD-10 in which a particular health condition is classified with a single code. As the functioning of a person can be affected at the body, individual and societal level, the user should always take into consideration all components of the classification, namely Body Functions and Structures, Activities and Participation, and Environmental Factors. Though it is impractical to expect that all the possible codes will be used for every encounter, depending on the setting of the encounter users will select the most salient codes for their purpose to describe a given health experience.

Code relevant information

Coded information is always in the context of a health condition. Although to use the codes it is not necessary to trace the links between the health condition and the aspects of functioning and disability that are coded, ICF is a health classification and so presumes the presence of a health condition of some kind. Therefore, information about what a person does or does not choose to do is not related to a functioning problem associated with a health condition and should not be coded. For example, if a person decides not to begin new relationships with his or her neighbours for reasons other than health, then it is not appropriate to use category d7200, which includes the actions of forming relationships. Conversely, if the person's decision is linked to a health condition (e.g. depression), then the code should be applied.

Information that reflects the person's feeling of involvement or satisfaction with the level of functioning is currently not coded in ICF. Further research may provide additional qualifiers that will allow this information to be coded.

Only those aspects of the person's functioning relevant to a predefined time-frame should be coded. Functions that relate to an earlier encounter and have no bearing on the current encounter should not be recorded.

Code explicit information

When assigning codes, the user should not make an inference about the inter-relationship between an impairment of body functions or structure, activity limitation or participation restriction. For example, if a person has a limitation in functioning in moving around, it is not justifiable to assume that the person has an impairment of movement functions. Similarly, from the fact that a person has a limited capacity to move around it is unwarranted to infer that he or she has a performance problem in moving around. The user must obtain explicit information on Body Functions and Structures and on capacity and performance separately (in some instances, mental functions for example, an inference from other observations is required since the body function in question is not directly observable).

Code specific information

Health and health-related states should be recorded as specifically as possible, by assigning the most appropriate ICF category. For example, the most specific code for a person with night blindness is b21020 "Light sensitivity". If, however, for some reason this level of detail cannot be applied, the corresponding "parent" code in the hierarchy can be used instead (in this case, b2102 Quality of vision, b210 Seeing functions, or b2 Sensory functions and pain).

To identify the appropriate code easily and quickly, the use of the ICF Browser,[12] which provides a search engine function with an electronic index of the full version of the classification, is strongly recommended. Alternatively, the alphabetical index can be used.

3. Coding conventions for the Environmental Factors component

For the coding of environmental factors, three coding conventions are open for use:

Convention 1

Environmental factors are coded alone, without relating these codes to body functions, body structures or activities and participation.

Body functions	_____
Body structures	_____
Activities and Participation	_____
Environment	_____

Convention 2

Environmental factors are coded for every component.

Body functions	_____	E code _____
Body structures	_____	E code _____
Activities and Participation	_____	E code _____

---

[12] The ICF Browser in different languages can be downloaded from the ICF website: http://www.who.int/classification/icf

Convention 3

Environmental factors are coded for capacity and performance qualifiers in the Activities and Participation component for every item.

Performance qualifier_____   E code _____
Capacity qualifier _____   E code _____

4. Component-specific coding rules

4.1 Coding body functions

Definitions

Body functions are the physiological functions of body systems (including psychological functions). *Impairments* are problems in body function or structure as a significant deviation or loss.

Using the qualifier for body functions

Body functions are coded with one qualifier that indicates the extent or magnitude of the impairment. The presence of an impairment can be identified as a loss or lack, reduction, addition or excess, or deviation.

The impairment of a person with hemiparesis can be described with code b7302 Power of muscles of one side of the body:

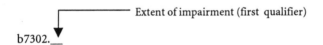

Extent of impairment (first qualifier)

b7302.__

Once an impairment is present, it can be scaled in severity using the generic qualifier. For example:

b7302.1 MILD impairment of power of muscles of one side of body   (5–24 %)
b7302.2 MODERATE impairment of power of muscles of one side of body   (25–49 %)
b7302.3 SEVERE impairment of power of muscles of one side of body   (50–95 %)
b7302.4 COMPLETE impairment of power of muscles of one side of body   (96–100 %)

The absence of an impairment (according to a predefined threshold level) is indicated by the value "0" for the generic qualifier. For example:

b7302.0 NO impairment in power of muscles of one side of body

If there is insufficient information to specify the severity of the impairment, the value "8" should be used. For example, if a person's health record states that the person is suffering from weakness of the right side of the body without giving further details, then the following code can be applied:

b7302.8 Impairment of power of muscles of one side of body, not specified

There may be situations where it is inappropriate to apply a particular code. For example, the code b650 Menstruation functions is not applicable for women before or beyond a certain age (pre-menarche or post-menopause). For these cases, the value "9" is assigned:

b650.9 Menstruation functions, not applicable

Structural correlates of body functions

The classifications of Body Functions and Body Structures are designed to be parallel. When a body function code is used, the user should check whether the corresponding body structure code is applicable. For example, body functions include basic human senses such as b210-b229 Seeing and related functions," and their structural correlates occur between s210 and s230 as "eye and related structures" .

Interrelationship between impairments

Impairments may result in other impairments; for example, muscle power may impair movement functions, heart functions may relate to respiratory functions, perception may relate to thought functions.

Identifying impairments in body functions

For those impairments that cannot always be observed directly (e.g. mental functions), the user can infer the impairment from observation of behaviour. For example, in a clinical setting memory may be assessed through standardized tests, and although it is not possible to actually "observe" brain function, depending on the results of these tests it may be reasonable to assume that the mental functions of memory are impaired.

4.2 Coding body structures

Definitions

Body structures are anatomical parts of the body such as organs, limbs and their components. **Impairments** are problems in body function or structure as a significant deviation or loss.

Using qualifiers for coding body structures

Body structures are coded with three qualifiers. The first qualifier describes the extent or magnitude of the impairment, the second qualifier is used to indicate the nature of the change, and the third qualifier denotes the location of the impairment.

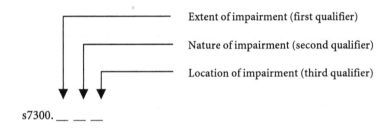

Extent of impairment (first qualifier)

Nature of impairment (second qualifier)

Location of impairment (third qualifier)

s7300. __ __ __

The descriptive schemes used for the three qualifiers are listed in Table 1.

Table 1. Scaling of qualifiers for body structures

First qualifier Extent of impairment	Second qualifier Nature of impairment	Third qualifier (suggested) Location of impairment
0 NO impairment 1 MILD impairment 2 MODERATE impairment 3 SEVERE impairment 4 COMPLETE impairment 8 not specified 9 not applicable	0 no change in structure 1 total absence 2 partial absence 3 additional part 4 aberrant dimensions 5 discontinuity 6 deviating position 7 qualitative changes in structure, including accumulation of fluid 8 not specified 9 not applicable	0 more than one region 1 right 2 left 3 both sides 4 front 5 back 6 proximal 7 distal 8 not specified 9 not applicable

4.3 Coding the Activities and Participation component

Definitions
Activity is the execution of a task or action by an individual. *Participation* is involvement in a life situation. *Activity limitations* are difficulties an individual may have in executing activities. *Participation restrictions* are problems an individual may experience in involvement in life situations.

The Activities and Participation classification is a single list of domains.

Using the capacity and performance qualifiers
Activities and Participation is coded with two qualifiers: the *performance* qualifier, which occupies the first digit position after the point, and the *capacity* qualifier, which occupies the second digit position after the point. The code that identifies the category from the Activities and Participation list and the two qualifiers form the default information matrix.

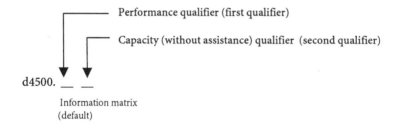

The performance qualifier describes what an individual does in his or her current environment. Because the current environment brings in a societal context, performance as recorded by this qualifier can also be understood as "involvement in a life situation" or "the lived experience" of people in the actual context in which they live. This context includes the environmental factors – i.e. all aspects of the physical, social and attitudinal world. This features of the current environment can be coded using the Environmental Factors classification.

The capacity qualifier describes an individual's ability to execute a task or an action. This construct aims to indicate the highest probable level of functioning that a person may reach in a given domain at a given moment. To assess the full ability of the individual, one would need to have a "standardized" environment to neutralize the varying impact of different environments on the ability of the individual. This standardized environment may be: (a) an actual environment commonly used for capacity assessment in test settings; (b) in cases where this is not possible, an assumed environment which can be thought to have an uniform impact. This environment can be called the "uniform" or "standard" environment. Thus, the capacity construct reflects the environmentally adjusted ability of the individual. This adjustment has to be the same for all persons in all countries to allow international comparisons. To be precise, the features of the uniform or standard environment can be coded using the Environmental Factors component. The gap between capacity and performance reflects the difference between the impacts of the current and uniform environments and thus provides a useful guide as to what can be done to the environment of the individual to improve performance.

Typically, the capacity qualifier without assistance is used in order to describe the individual's true ability which is not enhanced by an assistance device or personal assistance. Since the performance qualifier addresses the individual's current environment, the presence of assistive devices or personal assistance or barriers can be directly observed. The nature of the facilitator or barrier can be described using the Environmental Factors classification.

Optional qualifiers

The third and fourth (optional) qualifiers provide users with the possibility of coding capacity with assistance and performance without assistance.

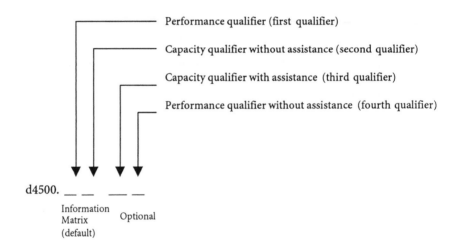

Performance qualifier (first qualifier)

Capacity qualifier without assistance (second qualifier)

Capacity qualifier with assistance (third qualifier)

Performance qualifier without assistance (fourth qualifier)

d4500. __ __   __ __

Information Matrix (default)   Optional

Additional qualifiers

The fifth digit position is reserved for qualifiers that may be developed in the future, such as a qualifier for involvement or subjective satisfaction.

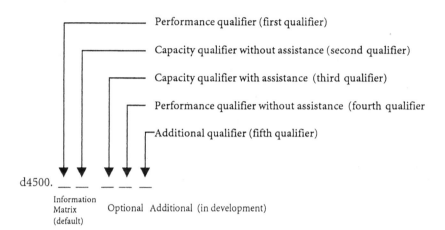

d4500. __ __ __ __ __

Information
Matrix   Optional Additional (in development)
(default)

Both capacity and performance qualifiers can further be used both with and without assistive devices or personal assistance, and in accordance with the following scale (where xxx stands for the second-level domain number):

     xxx.0 NO difficulty
     xxx.1 MILD difficulty
     xxx.2 MODERATE difficulty
     xxx.3 SEVERE difficulty
     xxx.4 COMPLETE difficulty
     xxx.8 not specified
     xxx.9 not applicable

When to use the performance qualifier and the capacity qualifier

Either qualifier may be used for each of the categories listed. But the information conveyed in each case is different. When both qualifiers are used, the result is an aggregation of two constructs, i.e.:

                                 d4500. 2 _

d4500. 2 1   ⟶

                                 d4500._ 1

If only one qualifier is used, then the unused space should not be filled with .8 or .9, but left blank, since both of these are true assessment values and would imply that the qualifier is being used.

Examples of the application of the two qualifiers

d4500 Walking short distances

For the *performance qualifier*, this domain refers to getting around on foot, in the person's current environment, such as on different surfaces and conditions, with the use of a cane, walker, or other assistive technology, for distances less than 1 km. For example, the performance of a person who lost his leg in a work-related accident and since then has used a cane but faces moderate difficulties in walking around because the sidewalks in the neighbourhood are very steep and have a very slippery surface can be coded:

d4500.3 _ moderate restriction in performance of walking short distances

For the *capacity qualifier*, this domain refers to the an individual's ability to walk around without assistance. In order to neutralize the varying impact of different environments, the ability may be assessed in a "standardized" environment. This standardized environment may be: (a) an actual environment commonly used for capacity assessment in test settings; or (b) in cases where this is not possible, an assumed environment which can be thought to have an uniform impact. For example, the true ability of the above-mentioned person to walk without a cane in a standardized environment (such as one with flat and non-slippery surfaces) will be very limited. Therefore the person's capacity may be coded as follows:

d4500._ 3 severe capacity limitation in walking short distances

Users who wish to specify the current or standardized environment while using the performance or capacity qualifier should use the Environmental Factors classification (see coding convention 3 for Environmental Factors in section 3 above).

4.4 Coding environmental factors

Definitions
Environmental Factors make up the physical, social and attitudinal environment in which people live and conduct their lives.

Use of Environmental Factors
Environmental Factors is a component of Part 2 (Contextual Factors) of the classification. Environmental factors must be considered for each component of functioning and coded according to one of the three conventions described in section 3 above.

Environmental factors are to be coded from the perspective of the person whose situation is being described. For example, kerb cuts without textured paving may be coded as a facilitator for a wheelchair user but as a barrier for a blind person.

The qualifier indicates the extent to which a factor is a facilitator or a barrier. There are several reasons why an environmental factor may be a facilitator or a barrier, and to what extent. For facilitators, the coder should keep in mind issues such as the accessibility of a resource, and whether access is dependable or variable, of good or poor quality and so on. In the case of barriers, it might be relevant how often a factor hinders the person, whether the hindrance is great or small, or avoidable or not. It should also be kept in mind that an environmental factor can be a barrier either because of its presence (for example, negative attitudes towards people with disabilities) or its absence (for example, the unavailability of a needed service). The effects that environmental factors have on the lives of people with health conditions are varied and complex, and it is hoped that future research will lead to a better understanding of this interaction and, possibly, show the usefulness of a second qualifier for these factors.

In some instances, a diverse collection of environmental factors is summarized with a single term, such as poverty, development, rural or urban setting, or social capital. These summary terms are not themselves found in the classification. Rather, the coder should separate the constituent factors and code these. Once again, further research is required to determine whether there are clear and consistent sets of environmental factors that make up each of these summary terms.

First qualifier

The following is the negative and positive scale that denotes the extent to which an environmental factor acts as a barrier or a facilitator. Using a point alone denotes a barrier, whereas using the + sign instead denotes a facilitator, as indicated below:

xxx.0 NO barrier	xxx+0 NO facilitator
xxx.1 MILD barrier	xxx+1 MILD facilitator
xxx.2 MODERATE barrier	xxx+2 MODERATE facilitator
xxx.3 SEVERE barrier	xxx+3 SUBSTANTIAL facilitator
xxx.4 COMPLETE barrier	xxx+4 COMPLETE facilitator
xxx.8 barrier, not specified	xxx+8 facilitator, not specified
xxx.9 not applicable	xxx.9 not applicable

Annex 3

Possible uses of the Activities and Participation list

The Activities and Participation component is a neutral list of domains indicating various actions and life areas. Each domain contains categories at different levels ordered from general to detailed (e.g. the domain of Chapter 4 Mobility, contains categories such as d450 Walking and under it the more specific item, d4500 Walking short distances.) The list of activity and participation domains covers the full range of functioning, which can be coded at both the individual and societal levels.

As indicated in the Introduction, this list can be used in different ways to indicate the specific notions of "Activities" and "Participation", which are defined in ICF as follows:

> In the context of health:
>
> **Activity** is the execution of a task or action by an individual.
>
> **Participation** is involvement in a life situation.

There are four alternative options for structuring the relationship between activities (a) and participation (p) in terms of the domain list:

(1)   Distinct sets of ativities domains and participation domains (no overlap)

A certain set of categories is coded only as activities (i.e. tasks or actions that an individual does) and another set only as participation (i.e. involvement in life situations). The two sets, therefore, are mutually exclusive.

In this option, the sets of activity categories and participation categories is determined by the user. Each category is either an activity or a participation item, but not both. For example, the domains may be divided as follows:

a1 Learning and applying knowledge
a2 General tasks and demands
a3 Communication
a4 Mobility

                      p5 Self-care
                      p6 Domestic life
                      p7 Interpersonal interactions
                      p8 Major life areas
                      p9 Community, social and civic life

Coding for this structure

> a *category code.* q_p q_c (a category deemed an activities item)
>
> p *category code.* q_p q_c (a category deemed a participation item)

Where q_p = the performance qualifier and q_c = the capacity qualifier. If the performance qualifier is used, the category, whether denoted as an activities or a participation item, is interpreted in terms of the performance construct; if the capacity qualifier is used, a capacity construct is used to interpret the category, again whether denoted as an activities or a participation item.

In this way option (1) provides the full information matrix without any redundancy or overlap.

(2)   Partial overlap between sets of activities and participation domains

In this alternative, a set of categories may be interpreted as both activities and participation items; that is, the same category is thought to be open to an individual (i.e. as a task or action that an individual does) and a societal (i.e. involvement in a life situation) interpretation.

For example:

a1 Learning and applying knowledge	
a2 General tasks and demands	
a3 Communication	p3 Communication
a4 Mobility	p4 Mobility
a5 Self-care	p5 Self-care
a6 Domestic life	p6 Domestic life
	p7 Interpersonal interactions
	p8 Major life areas
	p9 Community, social and civic life

Coding for this structure

There is a restriction on how categories can be coded for this structure. It cannot be possible for a category within the "overlap" to have different values for the same qualifier (either the first qualifier for performance or the second qualifier for capacity), e.g.:

> a *category.* 1 _   or   a *category.* _ 1
> p *category.* 2   p *category.* _ 2

A user who chooses this option believes that codes in the overlapping categories may mean different things when they are coded in activities and not in participation, and vice versa. However, one single code has to be entered into the information matrix for the specified qualifier column.

(3)   Detailed categories as activities and broad categories as participation, with or without overlap

Another approach to applying activities and participation definitions to the domains restricts participation to the more general or broader categories within a domain (e.g. first-level categories such as chapter headings) and deems the more detailed categories to be activities (e.g. third- or fourth-level categories). This approach separates categories within some or all domains in terms of the broad versus detailed distinction. The user may deem some domains to be entirely (i.e. at all levels of detail) activities or entirely participation.

For example, d4550 Crawling may be construed as an activity while d455 Moving around may be construed as participation.

There are two possible ways of handling this approach: (a) there is no "overlap", i.e. if an item is an activity it is not participation; or (b) there may be an overlap, since some users may use the whole list for activities and only broad titles for participation.

Coding for this structure

Similar to option (1) or option (2).

(4)   Use of the same domains for both activities and participation with total overlap of domains

In this option, all domains in the Activities and Participation list can be viewed as both activities and participation. Every category can be interpreted as individual functioning (activity) as well as societal functioning (participation).

For example, d330 Speaking can be seen both as an activity and as participation. A person with missing vocal cords can speak with the use of an assistive device. According to the assessments using capacity and performance qualifiers, this person has:

> *First qualifier*
> Moderate difficulty in performance (perhaps because of contextual
> factors such as personal stress or other peoples', attitudes)   → 2

> *Second qualifier*
> Severe difficulty in capacity without assistive device   → 3

> *Third qualifier*
> Mild difficulty in capacity with assistive device   → 1

According to the ICF information matrix this person's situation should be coded as:

> d330.231

According to option (4) this can also be coded as:

a330.231
p330.2

In option (4), when both performance and capacity qualifiers are used, there are two values for the same cell in the ICF information matrix: one for activities and one for participation. If these values are the same, then there is no conflict, only redundancy. However, in the case of differing values, users must develop a decision rule to code for the information matrix, since the official WHO coding style is this:

d *category* q_p q_c

One possible way to overcome this redundancy may be to consider the capacity qualifier as activity and the performance qualifier as participation.

Another possibility is to develop additional qualifiers for participation that capture "involvement in life situations".

It is expected that with the continued use of ICF and the generation of empirical data, evidence will become available as to which of the above options are preferred by different users of the classification. Empirical research will also lead to a clearer operationalization of the notions of activities and participation. Data on how these notions are used in different settings, in different countries and for different purposes can be generated and will then inform further revisions to the scheme.

Annex 4

Case examples

The examples below describe applications of ICF concepts to various cases. It is hoped that they will assist users to understand the intent and application of the basic classification concepts and constructs. For further details, please refer to WHO training manuals and courses.

Impairment leading to no limitation in capacity and no problem in performance

A child is born with a fingernail missing. This malformation is an impairment of structure, but does not interfere with the function of the child's hand or what the child can do with that hand, so there is no limitation in the child's capacity. Similarly, there may be no performance problem – such as playing with other children without being teased or excluded from play –because of this malformation. The child, therefore, has no capacity limitations or problems in performance.

Impairment leading to no limitation in capacity but to problems in performance

A diabetic child has an impairment of function: the pancreas does not function adequately to produce insulin. Diabetes can be controlled by medication, namely insulin. When the body functions (insulin levels) are under control, there are no limitations in capacity associated with the impairment. However, the child with diabetes is likely to experience a performance problem in socializing with friends or peers when eating is involved, since the child is required to restrict sugar intake. The lack of appropriate food would create a barrier. Therefore, the child would have a lack of involvement in socialisation in the current environment unless steps were taken to ensure that appropriate food was provided, in spite of no limitations in capacity.

Another example is that of an individual with vitiligo on the face but no other physical complaints. This cosmetic problem produces no limitations in capacity. However, the individual may live in a setting where vitiligo is mistaken for leprosy and so considered contagious. In the person's current environment, therefore, this negative attitude is an environmental barrier that leads to significant performance problems in interpersonal interactions.

Impairment leading to limitations in capacity and – depending on circumstance – to problems or no problems in performance

A significant variation in intellectual development is a mental impairment. This may lead to some limitation in a variety of the person's capacities. Environmental factors, however, may affect the extent of the individual's performance in different life domains. For example, a child with this mental impairment might experience little disadvantage in an environment where expectations are not high for the general population and where the child is given an array of simple, repetitive but necessary tasks to accomplish. In this environment the child will perform well in different life situations.

A similar child growing up in an environment of competition and high scholastic expectation might experience more problems in performance in various life situations compared to the first child.

This case example highlights two issues. The first is that the population norm or standard against which an individual's functioning is compared must be appropriate to the actual current environment. The second is that the presence or absence of environmental factors may have either a facilitating or a hindering impact on that functioning.

Former impairment leading to no limitations in capacity but still causing problems in performance

An individual who has recovered from an acute psychotic episode, but who bears the stigma of having been a "mental patient", may experience problems in performance in the domain of employment or interpersonal interactions, because of negative attitudes of people in his or her environment. The person's involvement in employment and social life is, therefore, restricted.

Different impairments and limitations in capacity leading to similar problems in performance

An individual may not be hired for a job because the extent of his or her impairment (quadriplegia) is seen to preclude performing some job requirements (e.g. using a computer with a manual keyboard). The workplace does not have the necessary adaptations to facilitate the person's performance of these job requirements (e.g. voice recognition software that replaces the manual keyboard).

Another individual with less severe quadriplegia may have the capacity to do the necessary job tasks, but may not be hired because the quota for hiring people with disabilities has been filled.

A third individual, who is capable of performing the required job activities, may not be hired because he or she has an activity limitation that is alleviated through use of a wheelchair, although the job site is not accessible to wheelchairs.

Lastly, an individual using a wheelchair may be hired for the job, and has the capacity to do the job tasks and in fact does perform them in the work context. None the less, this individual may still have problems in performing in domains of interpersonal interactions with co-workers, because access to work-related rest areas is not available. This problem of performance in socializing at the place of employment may prevent access to job advancement opportunities.

All four individuals experience performance problems in the domain of employment because of different environmental factors interacting with their health condition or impairment. For the first individual, the environmental barriers include lack of accommodation at the workplace and probably negative attitudes. The second individual is faced with negative attitudes about employment of disabled people. The third person faces lack of accessibility of the built environment and the last person faces negative attitudes about disability generally.

Suspected impairment leading to marked problems in performance without limitations in capacity

An individual has been working with patients who have AIDS. This individual is otherwise healthy but has to undergo periodic testing for HIV. He has no capacity limitations. Despite this, people who know him socially suspect he may have acquired the virus and so avoid him. This leads to significant problems in the person's performance in the domain of social interactions and community, social and civic life. His involvement is restricted because of negative attitudes adopted by the people in his environment.

Impairments currently not classified in ICF leading to problems in performance

An individual has a mother who died of breast cancer. She is 45 years old and was voluntarily screened recently and found to carry the genetic code that puts her at risk for breast cancer. She has no problems in body function or structure, or limitation in capacities, but is denied health insurance by her insurance company because of her increased risk for breast cancer. Her involvement in the domain of looking after her health is restricted because of the policy of the health insurance company.

Additional examples

A 10-year-old boy is referred to a speech therapist with the referral diagnosis "stuttering". During the examination problems are found in discontinuities in speech, inter- and intra-verbal accelerations, problems in timing of speech movements and inadequate speech rhythm (impairments). There are problems at school with reading aloud and with conversation (capacity limitations). During group discussions he does not take any initiative to engage in the discussions although he would like to (performance problem in the domain of conversing with many people). This boy's involvement in conversation is limited when in a group because of societal norms and practices concerning the orderly unfolding of conversations.

A 40-year-old woman with a whiplash injury four months earlier complains about pain in the neck, severe headache, dizziness, reduced muscle power and anxiety (impairments). Her ability to walk, cook, clean, handle a computer and drive a car are limited (limitations in capacity). In consultation with her physician it was mutually agreed to wait till the problems are reduced before she can return to her old full-time fixed-hours job (problems in performance in the domain of employment). If the workplace policies in her current environment allowed for flexible work hours, taking time off when her symptoms were particularly bad, and allowed her to work from home, her involvement in the domain of employment would improve.

Annex 5

ICF and people with disabilities

The ICF revision process has, since its inception, benefited from the input of people with disabilities and organizations of disabled persons. Disabled Peoples' International in particular has contributed its time and energies to the process of revision, and ICF reflects this important input.

WHO recognizes the importance of the full participation of persons with disabilities and their organizations in the revision of a classification of functioning and disability. As a classification, ICF will serve as the basis for both the assessment and measurement of disability in many scientific, clinical, administrative and social policy contexts. As such, it is a matter of concern that ICF not be misused in ways that are detrimental to the interests of persons with disabilities (see Ethical Guidelines in Annex 6).

In particular, WHO recognizes that the very terms used in the classification can, despite the best efforts of all, be stigmatizing and labelling. In response to this concern, the decision was made early in the process to drop the term "handicap" entirely – owing to its pejorative connotations in English – and not to use the term "disability" as the name of a component, but to keep it as the overall, umbrella term.

There remains, however, the difficult question of how best to refer to individuals who experience some degree of functional limitation or restriction. ICF uses the term "disability" to denote a multidimensional phenomenon resulting from the interaction between people and their physical and social environment. For a variety of reasons, when referring to individuals, some prefer to use the term "people with disabilities" while others prefer "disabled people". In the light of this divergence, there is no universal practice for WHO to adopt, and it is not appropriate for ICF rigidly to adopt one rather than another approach. Instead, WHO confirms the important principle that people have the right to be called what they choose.

It is important to stress, moreover, that ICF is not a classification of people at all. It is a classification of people's health characteristics within the context of their individual life situations and environmental impacts. It is the interaction of the health characteristics and the contextual factors that produces disability. This being so, individuals must not be reduced to, or characterized solely in terms of, their impairments, activity limitations, or participation restrictions. For example, instead of referring to a "mentally handicapped person", the classification uses the phrase "person with a problem in learning ". ICF ensures this by avoiding any reference to a person by means of a health condition or disability term, and by using neutral, if not positive, and concrete language throughout.

To further address the legitimate concern of systematic labelling of people, the categories in ICF are expressed in a neutral way to avoid depreciation, stigmatization and inappropriate connotations. This approach, however, brings with it the problem of what might be called the "sanitation of terms". The negative attributes of one's health condition and how other people react to it are independent of the terms used to define the condition. Whatever disability is called, it exists irrespective of labels. The problem is not only an issue of language but also, and mainly, an issue of the attitudes of other individuals and society towards disability. What is needed is correct content and usage of terms and classification.

WHO is committed to continuing efforts to ensure that persons with disabilities are empowered by classification and assessment, and not disentitled or discriminated against.

It is hoped that disabled people themselves will contribute to the use and development of ICF in all sectors. As researchers, managers and policy-makers, disabled people will help to develop protocols and tools that are grounded in the ICF classifications. ICF also serves as a potentially powerful tool for evidence-based advocacy. It provides reliable and comparable data to make the case for change. The political notion that disability is as much the result of environmental barriers as it is of health conditions or impairments must be transformed, first into a research agenda and then into valid and reliable evidence. This evidence can bring genuine social change for persons with disabilities around the world.

Disability advocacy can also be enhanced by using ICF. As the primary goal of advocacy is to identify interventions that can improve levels of participation of people with disabilities, ICF can assist in identifying where the principal "problem" of disability lies, whether it is in the environment by way of a barrier or the absence of a facilitator, the limited capacity of the individual himself or herself, or some combination of factors. By means of this clarification, interventions can be appropriately targeted and their effects on levels of participation monitored and measured. In this way, concrete and evidence-driven objectives can be achieved and the overall goals of disability advocacy furthered.

Annex 6

Ethical guidelines for the use of ICF

Every scientific tool can be misused and abused. It would be naive to believe that a classification system such as ICF will never be used in ways that are harmful to people. As explained in Appendix 5, the process of the revision of ICIDH has included persons with disabilities and their advocacy organizations from the beginning. Their input has lead to substantive changes in the terminology, content and structure of ICF. This annex sets out some basic guidelines for the ethical use of ICF. It is obvious that no set of guidelines can anticipate all forms of misuse of a classification or other scientific tool, or for that matter, that guidelines alone can prevent misuse. This document is no exception. It is hoped that attention to the provisions that follow will reduce the risk that ICF will be used in ways that are disrespectful and harmful to people with disabilities.

Respect and confidentiality

(1) ICF should always be used so as to respect the inherent value and autonomy of individual persons.

(2) ICF should never be used to label people or otherwise identify them solely in terms of one or more disability categories.

(3) In clinical settings, ICF should always be used with the full knowledge, cooperation, and consent of the persons whose levels of functioning are being classified. If limitations of an individual's cognitive capacity preclude this involvement, the individual's advocate should be an active participant.

(4) The information coded using ICF should be viewed as personal information and subject to recognized rules of confidentiality appropriate for the manner in which the data will be used.

Clinical use of ICF

(5) Wherever possible, the clinician should explain to the individual or the individual's advocate the purpose of the use of ICF and invite questions about the appropriateness of using it to classify the person's levels of functioning.

(6) Wherever possible, the person whose level of functioning is being classified (or the person's advocate) should have the opportunity to participate, and in particular to challenge or affirm the appropriateness of the category being used and the assessment assigned.

(7) Because the deficit being classified is a result of both a person's health condition and the physical and social context in which the person lives, ICF should be used holistically.

Social use of ICF information

(8) ICF information should be used, to the greatest extent feasible, with the collaboration of individuals to enhance their choices and their control over their lives.

(9) ICF information should be used towards the development of social policy and political change that seeks to enhance and support the participation of individuals.

(10) ICF, and all information derived from its use, should not be employed to deny established rights or otherwise restrict legitimate entitlements to benefits for individuals or groups.

(11) Individuals classed together under ICF may still differ in many ways. Laws and regulations that refer to ICF classifications should not assume more homogeneity than intended and should ensure that those whose levels of functioning are being classified are considered as individuals.

Annex 7

Summary of the revision process

The development of ICIDH

In 1972, WHO developed a preliminary scheme concerning the consequences of disease. Within a few months a more comprehensive approach was suggested. These suggestions were made on two important principles: distinctions were to be made between impairments and their importance, i.e. their functional and social consequences, and these various aspects or axes of the data were to be classified separately in different fields of digits. In essence, this approach consisted of a number of distinct, albeit parallel, classifications. This contrasted with the traditions of ICD, wherein multiple axes (etiology, anatomy, pathology, etc.) are integrated in a hierarchical system occupying only a single field of digits. The possibility of assimilating these proposals into a scheme compatible with the principles underlying the structure of ICD was explored. At the same time, preliminary attempts were made to systematize the terminology applied to disease consequences. These suggestions were circulated informally in 1973, and help was solicited particularly from groups with a special concern in rehabilitation.

Separate classifications for impairments and handicaps were circulated in 1974 and discussions continued. Comments were collated and definitive proposals were developed. These were submitted for consideration by the International Conference for the Ninth Revision of the International Classification of Diseases in October 1975. Having considered the classifications, the Conference recommended its publication for trial purposes. In May 1976, the Twenty-ninth World Health Assembly took note of this recommendation and adopted resolution WHA29.35, in which it approved the publication, for trial purposes, of the supplementary classification of impairments and handicaps as a supplement to, but not as an integral part of, the International Classification of Diseases. Consequently, the first edition of ICIDH was published in 1980. In 1993, it was reprinted with an additional foreword.

Initial steps in the revision of ICIDH

In 1993, it was decided to begin a process of revision of ICIDH. The desiderata for the revised version, know provisionally as ICIDH-2, were as follows:

- it should serve the multiple purposes required by different countries, sectors and health care disciplines;

- it should be simple enough to be seen by practitioners as a meaningful description of consequences of health conditions;

- it should be useful for practice - i.e. identifying health care needs and tailoring intervention programmes (e.g. prevention, rehabilitation, social actions);

- it should give a coherent view of the processes involved in the consequences of health conditions such that the disablement process, and not just the dimensions of diseases/disorders, could be objectively assessed, recorded and responded to;

- it should be sensitive to cultural variations (be translatable, and be applicable in different cultures and health care systems);

- it should be usable in a complementary way with the WHO family of classifications.

Originally, the French Collaborating Centre was given the task of making a proposal on the Impairments section and on language, speech and sensory aspects. The Dutch Collaborating Centre was to suggest a revision of the Disability and locomotor aspects of the Classification and prepare a review of the literature, while the North American Collaborating Centre was to put forward proposals for the Handicap section. In addition, two task forces were to present proposals on mental health aspects and children's issues respectively. Progress was made at a ICIDH-2 revision meeting held in Geneva in 1996, an Alpha draft was collated incorporating the different proposals, and initial pilot testing was conducted. It was decided at the 1996 meeting that each collaborating centre and task force would now be concerned with the draft as a whole and no longer with their former individual areas for revision. From May 1996 to February 1997, the Alpha draft was circulated among collaborating centres and task forces, and comments and suggestions were collated at WHO headquarters. A list of basic questions, setting out the main issues related to the revision, was also circulated in order to facilitate the collection of comments.

The following topics were considered during the process of revision:

- The three-level classification, i.e. Impairments, Disabilities and Handicaps, had been useful and should remain. The inclusion of contextual/ environmental factors should be considered, although most proposals remained at the stage of theoretical development and empirical testing.

- Interrelations between I/D/H and an adequate relationship between them had been an issue for discussion. Many criticisms had pointed to the causal model underlying the 1980 version of ICIDH, the lack of change over time, and the unidirectional flow from impairment to disability to handicap. The revision process had suggested alternative graphic representations.

- ICIDH-1980 was difficult to use. Simplification for use was deemed necessary: the revision should tend towards simplification rather than towards the addition of detail.

- Contextual factors (external – environmental factors/ internal–personal factors): These factors, which were major components of the handicap process (as conceptualized in the 1980 version of ICIDH), should be

247

developed as additional schemes within the ICIDH. However, since social and physical factors in the environment and their relationship to Impairments, Disabilities and Handicaps were strongly culture-bound, they should not be a separate dimension within ICIDH. Nevertheless, it was considered that classifications of environmental factors might prove useful in the analysis of national situations and in the development of solutions at the national level.

- Impairments should reflect advances in knowledge of basic biological mechanisms.

- Cultural applicability and universality should be a major aim.

- Development of training and presentation materials was also a major aim of the revision process.

ICIDH-2 Beta-1 and Beta-2 drafts

In March 1997, a Beta-1 draft was produced which integrated the suggestions collected over the previous years. This draft was presented to the ICIDH revision meeting in April 1997. After incorporation of the meeting's decisions the ICIDH-2 Beta-1 draft was issued for field trials in June 1997. Based on all the data and other feedback collected as part of the Beta-1 field trials, a Beta-2 draft was written between January and April 1999. The resulting draft was presented and discussed at the annual meeting on ICIDH-2 in London in April 1999. After incorporation of the meeting's decisions, the Beta-2 draft was printed and issued for field trials in July 1999.

Field trials

The field trials of the Beta-1 draft were conducted from June 1997 to December 1998, and the Beta-2 field trials from July 1999 to September 2000.

The field tests elicited the widest possible participation from WHO Member States and across different disciplines, including sectors such as health insurance, social security, labour, education, and other groups engaged in classifying health conditions (using the International Classification of Diseases, the Nurses' Classification, and the International Standard Classification of Education-ISCED). The aim was to reach a consensus, through clear definitions that were operational. The field trials constituted a continuous process of development, consultation, feedback, updating and testing.

The following studies were conducted as a part of the Beta-1 and Beta-2 field trials:

- translation and linguistic evaluation;

- item evaluation;

- responses to basic question by consensus conferences and individuals;

- feedback from organizations and individuals;

- options testing;

- feasibility and reliability in case evaluations (live or case summaries);

- others (e.g. focus group studies)

The testing focused on cross-cultural and multisectoral issues. More than 50 countries and 1800 experts were involved in the field tests, which have been reported separately.

ICIDH-2 Prefinal version

On the basis of Beta-2 field trial data and in consultation with collaborating centres and the WHO Committee of Experts on Measurement and Classification, the Prefinal version of ICIDH-2 was drafted in October 2000. This draft was presented to a revision meeting in November 2000. Following incorporation of the meeting's recommendations the ICIDH-2 Prefinal version (December 2000) was submitted to the WHO Executive Board in January 2001. The final draft of ICIDH-2 was then presented to the Fifty-fourth World Health Assembly in May 2001.

Endorsement of the final version

After discussion of the final draft, with the title International Classification of Functioning, Disability and Health, the Health Assembly endorsed the new classification in resolution WHA54.21 of 22 May 2001. The resolution reads as follows:

The Fifty-fourth World Health Assembly,

1.   ENDORSES the second edition of the International Classification of Impairments, Disabilities and Handicaps (ICIDH), with the title International Classification of Functioning, Disability and Health, henceforth referred to in short as ICF;

2.   URGES Member States to use the ICF in their research, surveillance and reporting as appropriate, taking into account specific situations in Member States and, in particular, in view of possible future revisions;

3.   REQUESTS the Director-General to provide support to Member States, at their request, in making use of ICF.

Annex 8

Future directions for ICF

Use of ICF will largely depend on its practical utility: the extent to which it can serve as a measure of health service performance through indicators based on consumer outcomes, and the degree to which it is applicable across cultures so that international comparisons can be made to identify needs and resources for planning and research. ICF is not directly a political tool. Its use may, however, contribute positive input to policy determination by providing information to help establish health policy, promote equal opportunities for all people, and support the fight against discrimination based on disability.

Versions of ICF

In view of the differing needs of different types of users, ICF will be presented in multiple formats and versions:

Main classification

The two parts and their components in ICF are presented in two versions in order to meet the needs of different users for varying levels of detail:

The first version is a *full (detailed) version* which provides all levels of classification and allows for 9999 categories per component. However, a much smaller number of them have been used. The full version categories can be aggregated into the short version when summary information is required.

The second version is a *short (concise) version* which gives two levels of categories for each component and domain. Definitions of these terms, inclusions and exclusions are also given.

Specific adaptations

(a) Clinical use versions: These versions will depend on the use of ICF in different clinical application fields (e.g. occupational therapy). They will be based on the main volume for coding and terminology; however, they will provide further detailed information such as guidelines for assessment and clinical descriptions. They can also be rearranged for specific disciplines (e.g. rehabilitation, mental health).

(b) Research versions: In a similar way to the clinical versions, these versions will respond to specific research needs and will provide precise and operational definitions to assess conditions.

Future work

Given the multitude of uses and needs for ICF, it is important to note that WHO and its collaborating centres are conducting additional work to meet those needs.

ICF is owned by all its users. It is the only such tool accepted on an international basis. It aims to obtain better information on disability phenomena and functioning and build a broad international consensus. To achieve recognition of ICF by various national and international communities, WHO has made every effort to ensure that it is user-friendly and compatible with standardization processes such as those laid down by the International Organization for Standardization (ISO).

The possible future directions for development and application of ICF can be summarized as follows:

- promoting use of ICF at country level for the development of national databases;

- establishing an international data set and a framework to permit international comparisons;

- identification of algorithms for eligibility for social benefits and pensions;

- study of disability and functioning of family members (e.g. a study of third-party disability due to the health condition of significant others);

- development of a Personal Factors component;

- development of precise operational definitions of categories for research purposes;

- development of assessment instruments for identification and measurement;[23]

- providing practical applications by means of computerization and case-recording forms;

- establishing links with quality-of-life concepts and the measurement of subjective well-being;[24]

- research into treatment or intervention matching;

---

[23] Assessment instruments linked to ICF are being developed by WHO with a view to applicability in different cultures. They are being tested for reliability and validity. Assessment instruments will take three forms: a brief version for screening/case-finding purposes; a version for daily use by care-givers; and a long version for detailed research purposes. They will be available from WHO.

[24] Links with quality of life: It is important that there is conceptual compatibility between "quality of life" and disability constructs. Quality of life, however, deals with what people "feel" about their health condition or its consequences; hence it is a construct of "subjective well-being". On the other hand, disease/disability constructs refer to objective and exteriorized signs of the individual.

- promoting use in scientific studies for comparison between different health conditions;

- development of training materials on the use of ICF;

- creation of ICF training and reference centres worldwide.

- further research on environmental factors to provide the necessary detail for use in describing both the standardized and current environment.

Annex 9

Suggested ICF Data requirements for ideal and minimal health information systems or surveys

Body Functions and Structures	Chapter and code		Classification block or category
Vision	2	b210–b220	Seeing and related functions
Hearing	2	b230–b240	Hearing and vestibular functions
Speech	3	b310-b340	Voice and speech functions
Digestion	5	b510–b535	Functions of the digestive system
Bodily excretion	6	b610–b630	Urinary functions
Fertility	6	b640–b670	Genital and reproductive functions
Sexual activity	6	b640	Genital and reproductive health
Skin and disfigurement	8	b810–b830	Skin and related structures
Breathing	4	b440–b460	Functions of the respiratory system
Pain*	2	b280	Pain
Affect*	1	b152–b180	Specific mental functions
Sleep	1	b134	Global mental functions
Energy/vitality	1	b130	Global mental functions
Cognition*	1	b140, b144,b164	Attention, memory and higher–level cognitive functions
Activities and Participation			
Communication	3	d310–d345	Communication receiving – producing
Mobility*	4	d450–d465	Walking and moving
Dexterity	4	d430–d445	Carrying, moving and handling objects
Self-care*	5	d510–d570	Self-care
Usual activities*	6 and 8		Domestic life; Major life areas
Interpersonal relations	7	d730–d770	Particular interpersonal relationships
Social functioning	9	d910–d930	Community social and civic life

---

*Candidate items for a minimal list

Appendix 10

Acknowledgements

The development of ICF would not have been possible without the extensive
support of many people from different parts of the world who have devoted a
great amount of time and energy and organized resources within an international
network. While it may not be possible to acknowledge them all here, leading
centres, organizations and individuals are listed below.

WHO Collaborating Centres for ICF

Australia	Australian Institute of Health and Welfare, GPO Box 570, Canberra ACT 2601, Australia. Contact: Ros Madden.
Canada	Canadian Institute for Health Information, 377 Dalhousie Street, Suite 200, Ottawa, Ontario K1N9N8, Canada. Contact: Helen Whittome.
France	Centre Technique National d'Etudes et de Recherches sur les Handicaps et les Inadaptations (CTNERHI), 236 bis, rue de Tolbiac, 75013 Paris, France. Contact: Marc Maudinet.
Japan	Japan College of Social Work, 3-1-30 Takeoka, Kiyose-city, Tokyo 204-8555, Japan. Contact: Hisao Sato.
Netherlands	National Institute of Public Health and the Environment, Department of Public Health Forecasting, Antonie van Leeuwenhoeklaan 9, P.O. Box 1, 3720 BA Bilthoven, The Netherlands. Contacts: Willem M. Hirs, Marijke W. de Kleijn-de Vrankrijker.
Nordic countries	Department of Public Health and Caring Sciences, Uppsala Science Park, SE 75185 Uppsala, Sweden. Contact: Björn Smedby.
United Kingdom of Great Britain and Northern Ireland	National Health System Information Authority, Coding and Classification, Woodgate, Loughborough, Leics LE11 2TG, United Kingdom. Contacts: Ann Harding, Jane Millar.
USA	National Center for Health Statistics, Room 1100, 6525 Belcrest Road, Hyattsville MD 20782, USA. Contact: Paul J. Placek.

Task forces

International Task Force on Mental Health and Addictive, Behavioural, Cognitive, and Developmental Aspects of ICIDH, Chair: Cille Kennedy, Office of Disability, Aging and Long-Term Care Policy, Office of the Assistant Secretary for Planning and Evaluation, Department of Health and Human Services, 200 Independence Avenue, SW, Room 424E, Washington, DC 20201, USA. Co-Chair: Karen Ritchie.

Children and Youth Task Force, Chair: Rune J. Simeonsson, Professor of Education, Frank Porter Graham Child Development Center, CB # 8185, University of North Carolina, Chapel Hill, NC 27599-8185, USA. Co-Chair: Matilde Leonardi.

Environmental Factors Task Force, Chair: Rachel Hurst, 11 Belgrave Road, London SW1V 1RB, England. Co-Chair: Janice Miller.

Networks

La Red de Habla Hispana en Discapacidades (The Spanish Network). Coordinator: José Luis Vázquez-Barquero, Unidad de Investigacion en Psiquiatria Clinical y Social Hospital Universitario "Marques de Valdecilla", Avda. Valdecilla s/n, Santander 39008, Spain.

Council of Europe Committee of Experts for the Application of ICIDH, Council of Europe, F-67075, Strasbourg, France. Contact: Lauri Sivonen.

Nongovernmental organizations

American Psychological Association, 750 First Street, N.E., Washington, DC 20002-4242, USA. Contacts: Geoffrey M. Reed, Jayne B. Lux.

Disabled Peoples International, 11 Belgrave Road, London SW1V 1RB, England. Contact: Rachel Hurst.

European Disability Forum, Square Ambiorix, 32 Bte 2/A, B-1000, Bruxelles, Belgium. Contact: Frank Mulcahy.

European Regional Council for the World Federation of Mental Health (ERCWFM), Blvd Clovis N.7, 1000 Brussels, Belgium. Contact: John Henderson.

Inclusion International, 13D Chemin de Levant, F-01210 Ferney-Voltaire, France. Contact: Nancy Breitenbach

Rehabilitation International, 25 E. 21st Street, New York, NY 10010, USA. Contact: Judith Hollenweger, Chairman, RI Education Commission, Institute of

Special Education, University of Zurich, Hirschengraben 48, 8001 Zurich, Switzerland.

Consultants

A number of WHO consultants provided invaluable assistance in the revision process. They are listed below.

Elizabeth Badley

Jerome E. Bickenbach

Nick Glozier

Judith Hollenweger

Cille Kennedy

Jane Millar

Janice Miller

Jürgen Rehm

Robin Room

Angela Roberts

Michael F. Schuntermann

Robert Trotter II

David Thompson (editorial consultant)

Translation of ICF in WHO official languages

ICF has been revised in multiple languages taking English as a working language only. Translation and linguistic analysis have been integral part of the revision process. The following WHO collaborators have lead the translation, linguistic analyses, editorial review the WHO official languages. Other translations could be found on the WHO-web site: http://www.who.int/classification/icf.

Arabic

Translation and linguistic analysis:
Adel Chaker, Ridha Limem, Najeh Daly, Hayet Baachaoui, Amor Haji, Mohamed Daly, Jamil Taktak, Saïda Douki

Editorial review carried out by WHO/EMRO:
Kassem Sara, M. Haytham Al Khayat, Abdel Aziz Saleh

Chinese

Translation and linguistic analysis:
Qiu Zhuoying (co-ordinator), Hong Dong, Zhao Shuying, Li Jing, Zhang Aimin, Wu Xianguang, Zhou Xiaonan

Editorial review carried out by WHO Collaborating Centre in China and WHO/WPRO:
Dong Jingwu, Zhou Xiaonan and Y.C. Chong

French

Translation and linguistic analysis carried out by WHO Geneva:
Pierre Lewalle

Editorial review carried out by WHO Collaborating Centres in France and Canada:
Catherine Barral and Janice Miller

Russian

Translation and linguistic analysis:
G. Shostka (Co-ordinator), Vladimir Y. Ryasnyansky, Alexander V. Kvashin, Sergey A. Matveev, Aleksey A. Galianov

Editorial review carried out by WHO Collaborating Centre in Russia:
Vladimir K. Ovcharov

Spanish

Translation, linguistic analysis, editorial review by the Collaborating Centre in Spain in collaboration with La Red de Habla Hispana en Discapacidades (The Spanish Network) and WHO/PAHO:
J. L. Vázquez-Barquero (Co-ordinator), Ana Díez Ruiz, Luis Gaite Pindado, Ana Gómez Silió, Sara Herrera Castanedo, Marta Uriarte Ituiño, Elena Vázquez Bourgon Armando Vásquez, María del Consuelo Crespo, Ana María Fossatti Pons, Benjamín Vicente, Pedro Rioseco, Sergio Aguilar Gaxiola, Carmen Lara Muñoz, María Elena Medina Mora, María Esther Araujo Bazán, Carlos Castillo-Salgado, Roberto Becker, Margaret Hazlewood

Individual participants in the revision process

Argentina
Liliana Lissi
Martha Adela Mazas
Miguela Pico
Ignacio Saenz

Armenia
Armen Sargsyan

Australia
Gavin Andrews
Robyne Burridge
Ching Choi
Prem K. Chopra
Jeremy Couper
Elisabeth Davis
Maree Dyson
Rhonda Galbally
Louise Golley
Tim Griffin
Simon Haskell
Angela Hewson
Tracie Hogan
Richard Madden
Ros Madden
Helen McAuley
Trevor Parmenter
Mark Pattison
Tony M. Pinzone
Kate Senior
Catherine Sykes
John Taplin
John Walsh

Austria
Gerhard S. Barolin
Klemens Fheodoroff
Christiane Meyer-
Bornsen

Belgium
Françoise Jan
Catherine Mollman
J. Stevens
A. Tricot

Brazil
Cassia Maria Buchalla
E. d'Arrigo Busnello
Ricardo Halpern
Fabio Gomes
Ruy Laurenti

Canada
Hugh Anton
J. Arboleda-Florez
Denise Avard
Elizabeth Badley
Caroline Bergeron

Hélène Bergeron
Jerome E. Bickenbach
Andra Blanchet
Maurice Blouin
Mario Bolduc (deceased)
Lucie Brosseau
T.S. Callanan
Lindsay Campbell
Anne Carswell
Jacques Cats
L.S. Cherry
René Cloutier
Albert Cook
Jacques Côté
Marcel Côté
Cheryl Cott
Aileen Davis
Henry Enns
Gail Finkel
Christine Fitzgerald
Patrick Fougeyrollas
Adele Furrie
Linda Garcia
Yhetta Gold
Betty Havens
Anne Hébert
Peter Henderson
Lynn Jongbloed
Faith Kaplan
Ronald Kaplan
Lee Kirby
Catherine Lachance
Jocelyne Lacroix
Renée Langlois
Mary Law
Lucie Lemieux-Brassard
Annette Majnemer
Rose Martini
Raoul Martin-Blouin
Mary Ann McColl
Joan McComas
Barbara McElgunn
Janice Miller
Louise Ogilvie
Luc Noreau
Diane Richler
Laurie Ringaert
Kathia Roy
Patricia Sisco
Denise Smith
Ginette St Michel
Debra Stewart
Luz Elvira Vallejo
Echeverri
Michael Wolfson
Sharon Wood-Dauphinee
Nancy Young
Peter Wass

Colleen Watters

Chile
Ricardo Araya
Alejandra Faulbaum
Luis Flores
Roxane Moncayo de
Bremont
Pedro Rioseco
Benjamin Vicente

China
Zhang Aimin
Mary Chu Manlai
Hong Dong
Leung Kwokfai
Karen Ngai Ling
Wu Xuanguong
Qiu Zhuoying
Zhao Shuying
Li Jing
Tang Xiaoquan
Li Jianjun
Ding Buotan
Zhuo Dahong
Nan Dengkun
Zhou Xiaonan

Colombia
Martha Aristabal Gomez

Côte d'Ivoire
B. Claver

Croatia
Ana Bobinac-Georgievski

Cuba
Pedro Valdés Sosa
Jesús Saiz Sánchez
Frank Morales Aguilera

Denmark
Terkel Andersen
Aksel Bertelsen
Tora Haraldsen Dahl
Marianne Engberg
Annette Flensborg
Ane Fink
Per Fink
Lise From
Jette Haugbølle
Stig Langvad
Lars von der Lieth
Kurt Møller
Claus Vinther Nielsen
Freddy Nielsen
Kamilla Rothe Nissen
Gunnar Schiøler
Anne Sloth

Susan Tetler
Selena Forchhammer
Thønnings
Eva Wæhrens
Brita Øhlenschlæger

Ecuador
María del Consuelo
Crespo
Walter Torres Izquierdo

Egypt
Mohammed El-Banna

El Salvador
Jorge Alberto Alcarón
Patricia Tovar de
Canizalez

Ethiopia
Rene Rakotobe

Finland
Erkki Yrjankeikki
Markku Leskinen
Leena Matikka
Matti Ojala
Heidi Paatero
Seija Talo
Martti Virtanen

France
Charles Aussilloux
Bernard Azema
Jacques Baert
Serge Bakchine
Catherine Barral
Maratine Barres
Jean-Yves Barreyre
Jean-Paul Boissin
François Chapireau
Pascal Charpentier
Alain Colvez
Christian Corbé
Dr. Cyran
Michel Delcey
Annick Deveau
Serge Ebersold
Camille Felder
Claude Finkelstein
Anne-Marie Gallot
Pascale Gilbert
Jacques Houver
Marcel Jaeger
Jacques Jonquères
Jean-Claude Lafon
Maryvonne Lyazid
Joëlle Loste-Berdot
Maryse Marrière
Lucie Matteodo
Marc Maudinet
Jean-Michel Mazeaux
Pierre Minaire*(deceased)*
Lucien Moatti
Bertrand Morineaux

Pierre Mormiche
Jean-Michel Orgogozo
Claudine Parayre
Gérard Pavillon
André Philip
Nicole Quemada
Jean-François Ravaud
Karen Ritchie
Jean-Marie Robine
Isabelle Romieu
Christian Rossignol
Pascale Roussel
Jacques Roustit
Jésus Sanchez
Marie-José Schmitt
Jean-Luc Simon
Lauri Sivonen
Henri-Jacques Stiker
Annie Triomphe
Catherine Vaslin
Paul Veit
Dominique Velche
Jean-Pierre Vignat
Vivian Waltz

Germany
Helmi Böse-Younes
Horst Dilling
Thomas Ewert
Kurt Maurer
Jürgen Rehm
H.M. Schian
Michael F.
Schuntermann
Ute Siebel
Gerold Stucki

Greece
Venos Mavreas

Hungary
Lajos Kullmann

India
Javed Abidi
Samir Guha-Roy
K.S. Jacob
Sunanda Koli
S. Murthy
D.M. Naidu
Hemraj Pal
K. Sekar
K.S. Shaji
Shobha Srinath
T.N. Srinivasan
R. Thara

Indonesia
Augustina Hendriarti

**Iran (Islamic Republic
of)**
Mohamed M.R. Mourad

Israel
Joseph Yahav

Italy
Emilio Alari
Alberto Albanese
Renzo Andrich
A.Andrigo
Andrea Arrigo
Marco Barbolini
Maurizio Bejor
Giulio Borgnolo
Gabriella Borri
Carlo Caltagirone
Felicia Carletto
Carla Colombo
Francesca Cretti
Maria Cufersin
Marta Dao
Mario D'Amico
Simona Della Bianca
Paolo Di Benedetto
Angela Di Lorenzo
Nadia Di Monte
Vittoria Dieni
Antonio Federico
Francesco Fera
Carlo Francescutti
Francesca Fratello
Franco Galletti
Federica Galli
Rosalia Gasparotto
Maria Teresa Gattesco
Alessandro Giacomazzi
Tullio Giorgini
Elena Giraudo
Lucia Granzini
Elena Grosso
V. Groppo
Vincenzo Guidetti
Paolo Guzzon
Leo Giulio Iona
Vladimir Kosic
Matilde Leonardi
Fulvia Loik
Mariangela Macan
Alessandra Manassero
Domenico Manco
Santina Mancuso
Roberto Marcovich
Andrea Martinuzzi
Anna Rosa Melodia
Rosetta Mussari
Cristiana Muzzi
Ugo Nocentini
Emanuela Nogherotto
Roberta Oretti
Lorenzo Panella
Maria Procopio
Leandro Provinciali
Alda Pellegri
Barbara Reggiori
Marina Sala

Giorgio Sandrini
Antonio Schindler
Elena Sinforiani
Stefano Schierano
Roberto Sicurelli
Francesco Talarico
Gariella Tavoschi
Cristiana Tiddia
Walter Tomazzoli
Corrado Tosetto
Sergio Ujcich
Maria Rosa Valsecchi
Irene Vernero

Jamaica
Monica Bartley

Japan
Tsunehiko Akamatsu
Masataka Arima
Hidenobu Fujisono
Katsunori Fujita
Shinichiro Furuno
Toshiko Futaki
Hajime Hagiwara
Yuichiro Haruna
Hideaki Hyoudou
Takashi Iseda
Atsuko Ito
Shinya Iwasaki
Shizuko Kawabata
Yasu Kiryu
Akira Kodama
Ryousuke Matsui
Ryo Matsutomo
Yasushi Mochizuki
Kazuyo Nakai
Kenji Nakamura
Yoshukuni Nakane
Yukiko Nakanishi
Toshiko Niki
Hidetoshi Nishijima
Shiniti Niwa
Kensaku Ohashi
Mari Oho
Yayoi Okawa
Shuhei Ota
Fumiko Rinko
Junko Sakano
Yoshihiko Sasagawa
Hisao Sato
Yoshiyuki Suzuki
Junko Taguchi
Eiichi Takada
Yuji Takagi
Masako Tateishi
Hikaru Tauchi
Miyako Tazaki
Mutsuo Torai
Satoshi Ueda
Kousuke Yamazaki
Yoshio Yazaki

Jordan
Abdulla S.T. El-Naggar
Ziad Subeih

Kuwait
Adnan Al Eidan
Abdul Aziz Khalaf Karam

Latvia
Valda Biedrina
Aldis Dudins
Lolita Cibule
Janis Misins
Jautrite Karashkevica
Mara Ozola
Aivars Vetra

Lebanon
Elie Karam

Lithuania
Albinas Bagdonas

Luxembourg
Charles Pull
M. De Smedt
Pascale Straus

Malaysia
Sandiyao Sebastian

Madagascar
Caromène Ratomahenina
Raymond

Malta
Joe M. Pace

Mexico
Juan Alberto Alcantara
Jorge Caraveo Anduaga
María Eugenia Antunez
Fernando R. Jiménez
Albarran
Gloria Martinez Carrera
María-Elena Medina
Mora
Carmen E. Lara Muñoz

Morocco
Aziza Bennani

Netherlands
T. van Achterberg
Jaap van den Berg
A. Bloemhof
Y.M. van der Brug
R.D. de Boer
J.T.P. Bonte
J.W. Brandsma
W.H.E. Buntinx
J.P.M. Diederiks
M J Driesse
Silvia van Duuren-
Kristen
C.M.A. Frederiks

J.C. Gerritse
José Geurts
G. Gladines
K.A. Gorter
R.J. de Haan
J. Halbertsma
E.J. van der Haring
F.G. Hellema
C.H. Hens-Versteeg
Y. F. Heerkens
Y. Heijnen
W.M. Hirs
H. W. Hoek
D. van Hoeken
N. Hoeymans
C. van Hof
G.R.M. van Hoof
M. Hopman-Rock
A. Kap
E.J. Karel
Zoltan E. Kenessey
M.C.O. Kersten
M.W. de Kleijn-de
Vrankrijker
M.M.Y. de Klerk
M. Koenen
J.W. Koten
D.W.Kraijer
T. Kraakman
Guuss Lankhorst
W.A.L. van Leeuwen
P. Looijestein
H. Meinardi
W. van Minnen
A.E. Monteny
I. Oen
Wil Ooijendijk
W.J. den Ouden
R.J.M. Perenboom
A. Persoon
J.J. v.d. Plaats
M. Poolmans
F.J. Prinsze
C.D. van Ravensberg
K. Reynders
K. Riet-van Hoof
G. Roodbol
G.L. Schut
B. Stoelinga
M.M.L. Swart
L. Taal
H. Ten Napel
B. Treffers
J. Verhoef
A. Vermeer
J.J.G.M. Verwer
W. Vink
M. Welle Donker
Dirk Wiersma
J.P. Wilken
P.A. van Woudenberg
P.H.M. Wouters
P. Zanstra

Nicaragua
Elizabeth Aguilar
Angel Bonilla Serrano
Ivette Castillo
Héctor Collado
Hernández
Josefa Conrado
Brenda Espinoza
María Félix Gontol
Mirian Gutiérrez
Rosa Gutiérrez
Carlos Guzmán
Luis Jara
Raúl Jarquin
Norman Lanzas
José R. Leiva
Rafaela Marenco
María Alejandra
Martínez
Marlon Méndez
Mercedes Mendoza
María José Moreno
Alejandra Narváez
Amilkar Obando
Dulce María Olivas
Rosa E. Orellana
Yelba Rosa Orozco
Mirian Ortiz Alvarado
Amanda Pastrana
Marbely Picado
Susana Rappaciolli
Esterlina Reyes
Franklin Rivera
Leda María Rodríguez
Humberto Román
Yemira Sequeira
Ivonne Tijerino
Ena Liz Torrez
Rene Urbina
Luis Velásquez

Nigeria
Sola Akinbiyi
John Morakinyo
A. O. Odejide
Olayinka Omigbodun

Norway
Kjetil Bjorlo
Torbjorg Hostad
Kjersti Vik
Nina Vollestad
Margret Grotle Soukup
Sigrid Ostensjo

Pakistan
S. Khan
Malik H. Mubbashar
Khalid Saeed

Philippines
L. Ladrigo-Ignacio
Patria Medina

Peru
María Esther Araujo
Bazon
Carlos Bejar Vargas
Carmen Cifuentes
Granados
Roxana Cock Huaman
Lily Pinguz Vergara
Adriana Rebaza Flores
Nelly Roncal Velazco
Fernando Urcia
Fernández
Rosa Zavallos Piedra

Republic of Korea
Ack-Seop Lee

Romania
Radu Vrasti

Russia
Vladimir N. Blondin
Aleksey A. Galianov
I.Y. Gurovich
Mikhail V. Korobov
Alexander V. Kvashin
Pavel A. Makkaveysky
Sergey A. Matveev
N. Mazaeva
Vladimir K. Ovtcharov
S.V. Polubinskaya
Anna G. Ryabokon
Vladimir Y. Ryasnyansky
Alexander V. Shabrov
Georgy D. Shostka
Sergei Tsirkin
Yuri M. Xomarov
Alexander Y.
Zemtchenkov

Slovenia
Andreeja Fatur-Videtec

South Africa
David Boonzaier
Gugulethu Gule
Sebenzile Matsebula
Pam McLaren
Siphokazi Gcaza
Phillip Thompson

Spain
Alvaro Bilbao Bilbao
Encarnación Blanco
Egido
Rosa Bravo Rodriguez
María José Cabo
González
Marta Cano Fernández
Laura Cardenal Villalba
Ana Diez Ruiz
Luis Gaite Pindado
María García José
Ana Gómez Silió
Andres Herran Gómez

Sara Herrera Castanedo
Ismael Lastra Martinez
Marta Uriarte Ituiño
Elena Vázquez Bourgon
Antonio León Aguado
Díaz
Carmen Albeza Contreras
María Angeles Aldana
Berberana
Federico Alonso Trujillo
Carmen Alvarez Arbesú
Jesus Artal Simon
Enrique Baca Baldomero
Julio Bobes García
Antonio Bueno Alcántara
Tomás Castillo Arenal
Valentín Corces Pando
María Teresa Crespo
Abelleira
Roberto Cruz Hernández
José Armando De Vierna
Amigo
Manuel Desviat Muñoz
Ana María Díaz García
María José Eizmendi
Apellaniz
Antonio Fernández
Moral
Manuel A. Franco Martín
Luis Gaite Pinadado
María Mar García Amigo
José Giner-Ubago
Gregorio Gómez-Jarabo
José Manuel Gorospe
Arocena
Juana María Hernández
Rodríguez
Carmen Leal Cercos
Marcelino López Alvarez
Juan José Lopez-Ibor
Ana María López Trenco
Francisco Margallo Polo
Monica Martín Gil
Miguel Martín
Zurimendi
Manuel J. Martínez
Cardeña
Juan Carlos Miangolarra
Page
Rosa M.Montoliu Valls
Teresa Orihuela
Villameriel
Sandra Ortega Mera
Gracia Parquiña
Fernández
Rafael Peñalver
Castellano
Jesusa Pertejo
María Francisca Peydro
de Moya
Juan Rafael Prieto
Lucena

Miguel Querejeta
González
Miquel Roca Bennasar
Francisco Rodríguez
Pulido
Luis Salvador Carulla
María Vicenta Sánchez
de la Cruz
Francisco Torres
González
María Triquell Manuel
José Luis Vázquez-
Barquero
Miguel A.Verdugo
Alonso
Carlos Villaro Díaz-
Jiménez

Sweden
Lars Berg
Eva Bjorck-Akesson
Mats Granlund
Gunnar Grimby
Arvid Linden
Anna Christina Nilson
(deceased)
Anita Nilsson
Louise Nilunger
Lennart Nordenfelt
Adolf Ratzka
Gunnar Sanner
Olle Sjögren
Björn Smedby
Sonja Calais van
Stokkom
Gabor Tiroler

Switzerland
André Assimacopoulos
Christoph Heinz
Judith Hollenweger
Hans Peter Rentsch
Thomas Spuhler
Werner Steiner
John Strome
John-Paul Vader
Peter Wehrli
Rudolf Widmer

Thailand
Poonpit Amatuakul
Pattariya Jarutat
C. Panpreecha
K. Roongruangmaairat
Pichai Tangsin

Tunisia
Adel Chaker
Hayet Baachaoui
A. Ben Salem
Najeh Daly
Saïda Douki
Ridha Limam
Mhalla Nejia

Jamil Taktak

Turkey
Ahmet Gögüs
Elif Iyriboz
Kultegin Ogel
Berna Ulug

United Arab Emirates
Sheika Jamila Bint Al-
Qassimi

**United Kingdom of
Great Britain and
Northern Ireland**
Simone Aspis
Allan Colver
Edna Conlan
John E. Cooper
A. John Fox
Nick Glozier
Ann Harding
Rachel Hurst
Rachel Jenkins
Howard Meltzer
Jane Millar
Peter Mittler
Martin Prince
Angela Roberts
G. Stewart
Wendy Thorne
Andrew Walker
Brian Williams

**United States of
America**
Harvey Abrams
Myron J. Adams
Michelle Adler
Sergio A. Aguilor-Gaxiola
Barbara Altman
Alicia Amate
William Anthony
Susan Spear Basset
Frederica Barrows
Mark Battista
Robert Battjes
Barbara Beck
Karin Behe
Cynthia D. Belar
J.G. Benedict
Stanley Berent
Linas Bieliauskas
Karen Blair
F. Bloch
Felicia Hill Briggs
Edward P. Burke
Larry Burt
Shane S. Bush
Glorisa Canino
Jean Campbell
Scott Campbell Brown
John A. Carpenter
Christine H. Carrington

Judi Chamberlin
LeeAnne Carrothers
Mary Chamie
Cecelia B. Collier
William Connors
John Corrigan
Dale Cox
M. Doreen Croser
Eugene D'Angelo
Gerben DeJong
Jeffrey E. Evans
Timothy G. Evans
Debbie J. Farmer
Michael Feil
Manning Feinleib
Risa Fox
Carol Frattali
Bill Frey
E. Fuller
Cheryl Gagne
J. Luis Garcia Segura
David W. Gately
Carol George
Olinda Gonzales
Barbara Gottfried
Bridget Grant
Craig Gray
David Gray
Marjorie Greenberg
Arlene Greenspan
Frederick Guggenheim
Neil Hadder
Harlan Hahn
Robert Haines
Laura Lee Hall
Heather Hancock
Nandini Hawley
Gregory W. Heath
Gerry Hendershot
Sarah Hershfeld
Sarah Hertfelder
Alexis Henry
Howard Hoffman
Audrey Holland
Joseph G. Hollowell Jr
Andrew Imparato
John Jacobson
Judith Jaeger
Alan Jette
J. Rock Johnson
Gisele Kamanou-Goune
Charles Kaelber
Cille Kennedy
Donald G. Kewman
Michael Kita *(deceased)*
Edward Knight
Pataricia Kricos
Susan Langmore
Mitchell LaPlante
Itzak Levav
Renee Levinson
Robert Liberman
Don Lollar

Peter Love
David Lozovsky
Perianne Lurie
Jayne B. Lux
Reid Lyon
Anis Maitra
Bob MacBride
Kim MacDonald-Wilson
Peggy Maher
Ronald Manderscheid
Kofi Marfo
Ana Maria Margueytio
William C. Marrin
John Mather
Maria Christina
Mathiason
John McGinley
Theresa McKenna
Christine McKibbin
Christopher J.
McLaughlin
Laurie McQueen
Douglas Moul
Peter E. Nathan
Russ Newman
Els R. Nieuwenhuijsen
Joan F. van Nostrand
Jean Novak
Patricia Owens
Alcida Perez de
Velasquez
D. Jesse Peters
David B. Peterson
Harold Pincus
Paul Placek
Thomas E. Preston
Maxwell Prince
Jeffrey Pyne
Louis Quatrano
Juan Ramos
Geoffrey M. Reed
Anne Riley
Gilberto Romero
Patricia Roberts-Rose
Mark A. Sandberg
Judy Sangl
Marian Scheinholtz
Karin Schumacher
Katherine D. Seelman
Raymond Seltser
Rune J. Simeonsson
Debra Smith
Gretchen Swanson
Susan Stark
Denise G. Tate
Travis Threats
Cynthia Trask
Robert Trotter II
R. Alexander Vachon
Maureen Valente
Paolo del Vecchio
Lois Verbrugge

Katherine Verdolini
Candace Vickers
Gloriajean Wallace
Robert Walsh
Seth A. Warshausky
Paul Weaver
Patricia Welch
Gale Whiteneck
Tyler Whitney
Brian Williams
Jan Williams
Linda Wornall
J. Scott Yaruss
Ilene Zeitzer
Louise Zingeser

Uruguay
Paulo Alterway
Marta Barera
Margot Barrios
Daniela Bilbao
Gladys Curbelo
Ana M. Frappola
Ana M. Fosatti Pons
Angélica Etcheñique
Rosa Gervasio
Mariela Irigoin
Fernando Lavie
Silvia Núñez
Rossana Pipplol
Silvana Toledo

Vietnam
Nguyen Duc Truyen

Zimbabwe
Jennifer Jelsma
Dorcas Madzivire
Gillian Marks
Jennifer Muderedzi
Useh Ushotanefe

Organisations of the United Nations system

International Labour Organization (ILO)
Susan Parker

United Nations Children's Fund (UNICEF)
Habibi Gulbadan

United Nations Statistical Division
Margarat Mbogoni
Joann Vanek

United Nations Statistical Institute for Asia and the Pacific
Lau Kak En

United Nations Economic and Social Commission for Asia and Pacific
Bijoy Chaudhari

World Health Organization

Regional Offices

Africa: C. Mandlhate

Americas (Pan American Health Organisation): Carlos Castillo-Salgado, Roberto Becker, Margaret Hazlewood, Armando Vázquez

Eastern Mediterranean: A. Mohit, Abdel Aziz Saleh, Kassem Sara, M. Haytham Al Khayat

Europe: B. Serdar Savas, Anatoli Nossikov

South-East Asia: Than Sein, Myint Htwe

Western Pacific: R. Nesbit, Y.C. Chong

Headquarters

Various departments at WHO headquarters were involved in the revision process. Individual staff members who contributed to the revision process are listed belowwith their departments are listed below.

M. Argandoña, formerly of Department of Substance Abuse

Z. Bankowski, Council for International Organizations of Medical Sciences

J.A. Costa e Silva, formerly Division of Mental Health and Prevention of Substance Abuse

S. Clark, Department of Health Information, Management and Dissemination

C. Djeddah, Department of Injuries and Violence Prevention

A. Goerdt, formerly of Department of Health Promotion

M. Goracci, formerly of Department of Injury Prevention and Rehabilitation

M. A. Jansen, formerly of Department of Mental Health and Substance Dependence

A. L'Hours, Global Programme on Evidence for Health Policy

A. Lopez, Global Programme on Evidence for Health Policy

J. Matsumoto, Department of External Cooperation and Partnerships

C. Mathers, Global Programme on Evidence for Health Policy

C. Murray, Global Programme on Evidence for Health Policy

H. Nabulsi, formerly of IMPACT

E. Pupulin, Department of Management of Noncommunicable Diseases

C. Romer, Department of Injuries and Violence Prevention

R. Sadana, Global Programme on Evidence for Health Policy

B. Saraceno, Department of Mental Health and Substance Dependence

A. Smith, Department of Management of Noncommunicable Diseases

J. Salomon, Global Programme on Evidence for Health Policy

M. Subramanian, formerly of World Health Reporting

M. Thuriaux, formerly of Division of Emerging and other Communicable Diseases

B. Thylefors, formerly of Department of Disability/Injury Prevention and Rehabilitation

M. Weber, Department of Child and Adolescent Health and Development

Sibel Volkan and Grazia Motturi provided administrative and secretarial support.

Can Çelik, Pierre Lewalle, Matilde Leonardi, Senda Bennaissa and Luis Prieto carried out specific aspects of the revision work.

Somnath Chatterji, Shekhar Saxena, Nenad Kostanjsek and Margie Schneider carried out the revision based on all the inputs received.

T. Bedirhan Üstün managed and coordinated the revision process and the overall ICF project.

ICF

Index

Note: This index is provided as a general tool for accessing categories within the classifications and discussions of issues and key terms in the Introduction and Annexes. Only words and phrases actually found in the ICF are indexed here. It is hoped that a more complete index of the ICF will be separately published and include more extensive cross-references to the items found in the classification. Towards that end, WHO welcomes suggestions from users for terms and phrases that could be added to the index to increase its usefulness.